THE TWO FACES OF CANCER

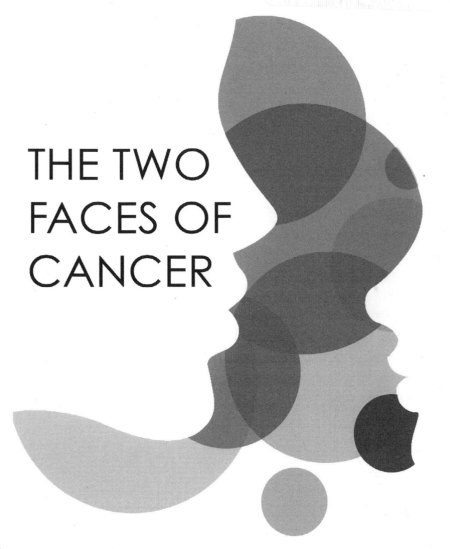

THE TWO FACES OF CANCER

Rebecca Brazier

Matador
9 Priory Business Park,
Wistow Road, Kibworth Beauchamp,
Leicestershire. LE8 0RX
Tel: 0116 279 2299
Email: books@troubador.co.uk
Web: www.troubador.co.uk/matador
Twitter: @matadorbooks

ISBN 978 1789014 822

British Library Cataloguing in Publication Data.
A catalogue record for this book is available from the British Library.

Printed and bound in the UK by TJ International, Padstow, Cornwall
Typeset in 12pt Minion Pro by Troubador Publishing Ltd, Leicester, UK

Matador is an imprint of Troubador Publishing Ltd

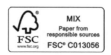

To Kate G
The person I never had and who showed me what it should have been like. Her care healed me and gave me the courage to be the person I was meant to be.

CONTENTS

Part II

ACKNOWLEDGEMENTS

There are many people to whom I am grateful for being there personally or professionally while I wrote this book; my oncologist who saved my life, Kate M for her numerous articles and unfailing support, Ian for his never-ending brilliant ideas and my editors for their helpful feedback. I would also like to thank the people who inspired me to write this book, and who believed in me, as well as the people who made me feel angry and then passionate enough to try and change something for cancer patients. Finally, an especially big thank you to my two awesome daughters, Poppy and Bonnie, who have been my reason to live when I wanted to give up and when it felt too tough to go on because, quite simply, I don't want to ever have to say goodbye to them.

INTRODUCTION

*"Only when we face the impossible, and experience the
unbearable, do we find out who we truly are."*

Vironika Tugaleva

How do you recover from the emotional impact of
cancer? This is a question most people who have been
diagnosed with cancer will have asked themselves. I
hope to answer that question by creating understanding
about the impact cancer has. I have written this book from
two perspectives, my three personal experiences of cancer
and my professional knowledge as a counsellor. The text
written in italics explains what happened to me from a
counselling perspective using basic counselling terms
which are referenced and explained at the end of the book.

We are all unique individuals who experience the
world in our own unique and individual way. Each cancer
diagnosis is as unique as the person being diagnosed and

we will each recover from cancer differently. I hope this book helps you understand your unique experience of cancer and that understanding helps you discover your way to recover.

Cancer was both the best and worst thing which ever happened to me. I love what it taught me and I loathe what it took. I liken it to a dandelion seed powerless in a strong wind, being blown away from all that is safe and familiar, to a far-off land. To a land where you know no one and no one knows you, and you have to start all over again having been bashed and beaten up on the way, having been dragged through raging rivers and across bleak, rocky mountain ranges. But this journey also creates clarity, purpose and a sharp and fresh perspective to life and living.

I hope this book inspires you to live your life fully.

PART I

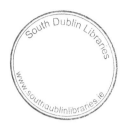

CHAPTER 1

"Motherhood changes everything."

Adriana Trigiani

This is my story of how one tiny cell caused so much chaos and change.

Let me introduce myself formally – I'm Rebecca, also known as Bex but never Becky, please never Becky. I was the firstborn in what turned out to be a large family in a large town in West Sussex. We argued frequently, plotted and executed dangerous activities, and I have wonderful memories of times with my three siblings. I've had my share of hangovers, exotic holidays, boring jobs and inappropriate relationships. I love fresh air, coastlines, woodlands, springtime, sunshine and wind. I loathe grey skies and rainy days. My favourite flowers are lilies and my favourite food is fruit. I get excited about bluebell woods. I hate offal and baked beans and don't watch soaps. I have never seen a Star Wars movie or read a Harry Potter book. I am rubbish at reversing and parallel parking. My favourite number is four. My favourite birds are swallows. My children's primary school values were Inspire, Achieve and Believe. These last three seemingly insignificant facts will have more meaning later on in the book.

I live in a tiny but beautiful hamlet on the Surrey/ Sussex border, with my husband Ian, our two daughters Poppy and Bonnie, a dog called Bo, two guinea pigs (names currently unknown as they keep being renamed), an escaped black rabbit, three ponies (Pandoe, Charly and Beanie) and some fish whose names no one can remember. We are surrounded by fields and trees, and have lovely friends close by. It sounds heavenly, doesn't it? But I also share my life with my unchosen, uninvited and unwanted lifelong companion, cancer.

Ian and I met in a pub in 1999. I was a waitress and he was a friend of one of the barmaids. He came in for a drink one Friday evening. I liked his cheeky smile, and he liked my thin legs. We got chatting and then dating, and then I moved in with him and gave up working in the pub. Ian was running a quantity surveying business; I was in the third year of a teaching degree. We lived in a semi-detached cottage with off-road parking and magnolia walls, at the end of a cul-de-sac in a quaint village. I loved horses and hated boats. He loved boats and hated horses. We were different but it worked; it was fun and at times a little crazy. We had a nice life and were settled. Time passed. We had been together for a couple of years and were in our mid-thirties.

From the age of twenty-three I had thought about being a mum but it never felt the right time or the right person and frequently it was neither. I still had no real urges to be a mum until one day out of the blue I asked myself how I would feel in ten years' time when at forty-six it would probably be too late. In that moment I knew I would regret not having children. Maybe this was the right time and the right person. We had a hasty conversation that evening about parenthood and casually began trying for a baby. We were made of fertile stuff and I got pregnant first time. When I saw the blue line on the pregnancy test I was both excited and terrified. My teaching degree instantly took a back seat and what was developing in me became my focus.

Within weeks our nice life had been replaced with morning sickness and weight gain. The morning sickness lasted well into the afternoon and evening. I felt sick constantly. I puked twice a day for four months. I would wake and drink a pint of water to dilute the bitter taste which was about to pass through my mouth at speed. I waited for a few moments until the familiar feelings appeared and I would run to the loo dreading what was about to happen. The only way to stop the constant nausea was to eat; ready meals did the trick. My thin legs soon became chunky.

Over the coming months my belly and its contents became my constant focus. I read countless pregnancy books and marvelled at the unseen which was developing daily inside of me. The second scan revealed we were expecting a girl. In that moment, I bonded with her and felt I was getting to know more about who was growing inside of me. I loved feeling and watching her kick and move around within me until she settled again. I was proud of my belly and its contents.

As first-time parents we did things just right. We researched, discussed and shopped on sunny Saturday afternoons for cots, car seats, mattresses, buggies, baths, nappies, muslins, blankets and all the other million things you think you need for a baby. We took an NCT course and designed our birth plan, which would of course be natural and drug-free. I packed my hospital bag and waited for the contractions to begin, flicking my way through baby name books and watching daytime TV.

At thirty-nine weeks a prenatal appointment revealed the precious cargo in my belly was positioned upside down and back to front. Options were discussed, all of which sounded unpleasant. I opted to have a Caesarean section and they had a space available the next day. Things sped up considerably at this point. I had about fourteen hours until I arrived at the hospital to become a mum. It's a good job I had already packed that hospital bag weeks ago and been so super-organised with my planning and shopping.

We left our village home early the next morning and arrived excitedly at the hospital. The hours ticked by, punctuated with visits from medical staff each of whom had a role to play over the coming hours. It was scorching hot. Eventually it was my turn and I was wheeled to the operating theatre, which was lit by bright lights. My belly looked like a huge dome under the white sheet. I met the surgical team and could hear clunking metal and medical terms being spoken around me. I lay still, paralysed from the legs down by an epidural. Ian reported back that the operation had begun and it was resembling something like a shark attack. It felt like rummaging for keys at the bottom of my handbag as Poppy Mae left my belly and entered this world. She became my world. Two became three. She was tiny, crumpled and beautiful. I was stitched up and we returned to the ward for a few days of monitoring, before being discharged to start my new role as a mum. I loved the visits by doting family members and texts from well-wishers as the news spread. I loved my new role and I loved her.

I blundered my way through being a new mum because beautiful, warm, tiny new bundles of joy don't arrive with an accompanying handbook or instruction leaflet. It was a shock to go from having exotic holidays and long lunches to days of feeling I had been successful if I had had my breakfast by 3pm and if I got dressed more than once a week. I still remember being woken at 3am on her first night in this world by a peculiar noise which I hadn't heard before. Very slowly I came to and realised it was a call for feed and then, very quickly, realised that it wasn't going to stop until I got up and fed her.

My boobs were now enormous. I wanted to breastfeed Poppy, but it hurt. I persevered. During the time I was feeding her I was diagnosed with and treated for mastitis twice. My left breast was red and inflamed and painful. Antibiotics did the trick. My ignorance and innocence was bliss. Having fed Poppy for six months I was knackered, well and truly knackered, but who isn't as a first-time mum? Isn't that what everyone tells you? I gradually stopped feeding her and began to purée organic carrots and broccoli, mix baby rice and mash bananas.

The floodgates of motherly love had been opened and I wanted more children, several in fact. I was heading to my late thirties and, having had a Caesarean section, I wanted to get cracking with number two as soon as possible. Around the end of January 2003 a thin blue line on a pregnancy test showed three was going to become four. This all seemed so easy and, thankfully, brought much less morning sickness. I would cope with a baby and toddler; it would all be just fine.

It was around this time, during an infrequent breast examination, I found a thickening in my depleted and now rather saggy post-breastfeeding left breast. There was no lump. It felt jagged around the edges. It wasn't there before. I did absolutely nothing about this discovery because thirty-eight-year-old pregnant women didn't get cancer, did they? And there was no lump. All the adverts say to look for a lump; a lump signals danger. This wasn't a lump.

I joined toddler and postnatal groups, making new friends and bonding through first-time motherhood. We whiled away the days talking baby stuff, reminiscing about our previous lives. We walked and swam, and chased crawling babies and then walking toddlers. We celebrated milestones; the first night they slept through and their first words. We comforted each other through their tantrums, vaccinations and illnesses.

> *The purpose and 'meaning' (page 322) to my life was now primarily defined as being a mother and I loved it. I felt loved and it was a privilege to love and care for this gorgeous and precious child. The other roles which I had previously had, such as student and employee, became less of a focus.*

We celebrated Poppy's first birthday with cake and balloons. We holidayed and had good times with friends and family. My thin legs and teaching degree seemed a lifetime ago. I was so tired, permanently. The pregnancy progressed normally and I waddled slowly everywhere in the summer heat with the lovely Poppy always close by my side. I loved holding her tiny hand in mine. The second scan revealed another girl, two sisters; how lovely, how perfect. I was already planning their matching outfits and the hats I would wear to their weddings. I was proud to update people and glowed with pride.

Around June, as my belly was getting bigger, the thickening in my breast was still there so I mentioned it casually to my matronly, and slightly scary, health visitor at an antenatal appointment. She felt the thickening and thought it was a blocked milk duct, which fitted nicely in my mind because of the mastitis. She suggested a daily massage to the area and, if it didn't go within a week, to see my GP.

The summer was hot and I was busy, so I did part of what she suggested, i.e. the massage, but I didn't visit the GP. My belly of baby grew; so did the unknown and undiagnosed tumour, spreading in its bid to break free and set up camp elsewhere in my body. It was only before the next visit to the matronly and the slightly scary health visitor, and with the thickening still there, that I visited my GP, out of fear of telling my matronly and slightly scary health visitor that I hadn't done what she had suggested. The GP examined me and also thought it was nothing but, to be on the safe side, referred me to our local hospital for further investigations, whatever that meant. During her examination she also found a large lump in my armpit. Still nothing remotely serious registered in my head and I was still totally ignorant of the fact that this had the potential to be anything serious.

The hospital appointment letter arrived a few days later. I casually read the letter and outline of the day. In my mind it would just be a swift appointment, merely a formality, and I would be home by lunchtime. I arranged care for Poppy and set off to the hospital appointment on my own because thirty-eight-year-old pregnant women didn't get cancer, did they?

My 'denial' (page 326) at the possibility of there being anything seriously wrong allowed me to engage with and enjoy my life as it was and protected me against the uncomfortable feelings of fear and anxiety.

CHAPTER 2

"If you're going through hell, keep going."

Winston Churchill

L ittle did I know as I woke up on this day, which is forever firmly engraved like a big and shiny brass plaque in my memory, that I was hours away from becoming a cancer patient; the day, the hour, the minute, the moment when the bomb goes off and nothing is ever the same again. An instant, full and lifelong membership of a club that no one wants to join and, once you are in, it's impossible to leave; no get-out clause or cooling-off period, returns or refund to your previous life. This day was 19th August 2003.

I was fortunate to have a 'one-stop clinic' at the hospital. Patients are seen by a consultant in the morning, have investigative tests during the day and return later for the results, like a day trip with a difference, where the activities are planned out for you. You meet new people, see different rooms, wear different outfits and experience several pieces of medical equipment. It was cleverly organised. First you meet with the breast care nurse, a lovely lady who takes some details and your name and address. This all seemed a bit irrelevant to me but I went along with the day's agenda. So far so good, I was still enjoying my pre-cancer diagnosis world. You then get to meet the consultant in the room next door. My thirty weeks of pregnant belly shuffled slowly and innocently from one room to the next. I felt out of place; shouldn't I be at the park with Poppy, feeding ducks stale bread and browsing the ice cream selection?

There sat the consultant, a spectacled and experienced surgeon. He rose from his seat to greet me with a handshake. The room was small and painted white and, although it was the height of summer, it felt cold with an impending feeling of doom. The room was cramped, there was an examination couch and a pile of worn hospital gowns in the corner next to a stack of neatly laundered ones. After a brief read of the breast care nurse's notes and a few quick questions, it was time to get my kit off and boobs out for an examination. It was now my turn to take a hospital gown from the neatly laundered pile and put it on and lie on the examination couch while the spectacled surgeon washed his hands. Things were turning slightly less amusing now.

The meaning of my breasts changed; no longer were they my husband's play things, producer of food for my children or something to make summer tops look good. They were now the focus of a medical examination, searching for health or ill health. The surgeon felt the thickening and I asked what he thought it was. Without eye contact he said I would need a biopsy (a biopsy takes a small piece of tissue to analyse what it is). What? Me? Are you sure? It all seemed a bit unnecessary. My pulse increased significantly and fear began to surge round my body. He gathered the medical kit needed and proceeded to take a fine needle biopsy. A fine needle (as the name suggests) was plunged into the thickening and a few cells were drawn off and sent for analysis. Only the needle isn't quite as fine as the name suggests. I was then referred for an ultrasound scan (an ultrasound scan uses high frequency sound waves to create an image) to gain more information about the thickening. I got down from the bed and threw my used gown on the pile with the others. He said he would see me later with the results. I dressed and took the form he had written on to radiography. I waddled along cool, soulless corridors following the signs. My day and my life were starting to unravel.

This was the first time during the eight weeks, from when I first mentioned the thickening to my matronly and slightly scary health visitor, that my thoughts changed – that this could be something serious – and they began surging at speed into my head along with the fear in my body. I was vaguely panicking; this kind of thing didn't happen to thirty-eight-year-old, thirty-week pregnant women, let alone me. I called Ian who came to the hospital, where he stayed with me for the rest of the day.

The unknown and uncertainty were creating anxiety and I asked Ian to come and support me, as in 'stage 1' (page 317). I could no longer remain in 'denial' (page 326) that there was nothing wrong. My feelings became more intense as the day progressed.

Ian, myself and my thirty-week pregnant belly returned at 5pm to a waiting room on a lower level in the hospital to receive the results of the biopsy and scan. Unbeknown to me I was now moments away from starting a lifelong connection with the wonderful world of oncology (oncology is a branch of medicine which treats cancer).

The orange walls created a surreal glow to the room. Magazines were scattered on the grey plastic chairs from the previous waits which had taken place throughout the day. I counted nine women in the waiting area. We sat in silence, each person deep in their own thoughts, each wondering what their next appointment would reveal. Each person was about to hear the results of their day's activities. I knew that statistically (at the time), a women has a one in nine lifetime risk of developing breast cancer and I wondered who here in this room of orange glow was going to be that person today.

I waited nervously, my heart pounding away in my chest just above where my baby was nesting, oblivious to what was living silently just above her. My name was called. My name was the first to be called. I entered the room and sat down apprehensively. The breast care nurse was also there. That's nice I thought. She sat perpendicular to the spectacled surgeon who sat behind a cheap, ugly, brown desk. *Boom, boom, boom* went my heart.

Spectacled surgeon began speaking. Spectacled surgeon suggested the conversation was recorded. I consented without thought, my mind now racing at the same speed as my heart. My mouth was dry, my cheeks stuck to my teeth. An old-fashioned tape recorder began whirring. Spectacled surgeon announced the results were back and in a swift and very well-rehearsed manoeuvre turned his laptop to face me and said that the fine needle biopsy had showed C5 cells. Time slowed, and my heart beat faster. On the white screen was a Word document and in the Word document was a table; a table with neat rows and columns, neat rows and columns that cause life-changing chaos. My eyes frantically scanned the page until they found 'C5'. On the same row, in the next column to 'C5', was a heart-stopping, life-changing word. 'Malignant'. FUCK.

In that split second at 17.51 on Tuesday 19th August 2003, my life changed, irreversibly. In the hideous moment when I read the word 'malignant' I immediately and instantly left my body and the rest of the meeting was conducted with me as an observer holding on to the ceiling, Spiderman style, observing the actors below. It was safe up here but down there, below me, was dangerous and frightening. I clung desperately to my tiny patch of life as death and fear swirled below me. My dignity held a wobbly and fragile smile, a smile that hid the churning turmoil and fear now surging, with no escape route, at speed through my body. I wasn't going to be able to negotiate or smile myself out of this.

The cancer diagnosis was a 'trauma' (page 332) and so overwhelming that I literally left my body because I could not cope with what I was hearing. It made no sense and didn't fit with the life I knew. I had no coping strategy or reference point to create understanding or

feel safe. My 'be strong' driver (page 329) kept me
from being vulnerable emotionally during the rest of
the appointment and I pinned on a fake smile to hide
the trauma and turmoil within me.

I asked no questions. I spoke no words. I was paralysed by the word I had read. It shut down my senses and froze me in a new and frighteningly unfamiliar world. I was told I would be referred to an oncologist. 'Malignant' and 'oncologist' were words I had not encountered before; words which had no meaning, words which had no place in my life, words that should not be used about you when you are thirty-eight years old and thirty weeks pregnant. Thank you and goodbye. Spectacled surgeon had completed his work; I would be passed on to someone else. He had taken the biopsy and delivered the findings. A pastel-coloured leaflet was given to me explaining the bomb which had just exploded in my life. The tape was ejected from the tape recorder and we left the room, silent and speechless. I wanted to cry and be sick, but I didn't because I couldn't.

I can't remember much of the rest of the meeting or the day but I do remember the lovely breast care nurse's kindness and care as we left the room and walked along a corridor to another room to try and make sense of what had just happened. I could see her role throughout the day. It had been cleverly orchestrated; the gentle introduction and then being there when your previous life and all that you know is punched out of you in the moments after diagnosis. I later found out that two women received a diagnosis that day, two women in one clinic in one small hospital. When you multiply that up, in other clinics, in other towns and cities of the UK and around the world, the numbers become terrifying; the lives that irrevocably change in a moment, with a word.

I wonder how many lives have been changed and shattered within those walls. How many people have left the room and walked, stumbled, sobbed down the corridor, dazed and disorientated, with cancer now very firmly in their lives and bodies? I am still left shocked that the consultant didn't use the word 'cancer' with me. If he couldn't say the word, how could I?

Recalling this experience still haunts me. I woke up as a pregnant mum and went to bed as a cancer patient. All my other roles in life – mum, sister, daughter, auntie and friend – removed and deleted. I was now a cancer patient who was going to die a quick, painful, bald death having spent a lot of time throwing up. All I could think about was dying. I was going to die and that was that. How the fuck could this be sorted out? And what about the baby? I simultaneously was living with life and death in my body, separated by inches.

The 'loss' (page 325) of the 'meaning' (page 322) of my life and the 'trauma' (page 332) began in the hours after diagnosis.

We left the hospital in the early evening; it was still scorching hot. Poor Poppy, we had been gone for so long. We collected her and I looked into her gorgeous blue eyes with my eyes full of tears. She was only fourteen months old, beautiful, giggly and innocent. I hugged her hard.

We then began the emotional and exhausting task of telling our family and friends I had cancer. We were still reeling from the shock of the diagnosis ourselves, without being plunged into having to tell people and manage zillions of questions, let alone their shock about the diagnosis, prognosis, treatment and the baby. Who should I tell first and how? My family were on a summer break in Bournemouth and I was reluctant to call them and ruin their holiday with this upsetting news.

I didn't really sleep that night. I could make no sense of my new world. Fear, panic and anxiety filled my days and nights. A tornado of thoughts and feelings cycled constantly. Flowers and cards arrived, and the calls and questions kept coming. How the fuck was this happening to me? I was so torn between wanting to live and wanting the best for my baby and was unsure if the two would be compatible. It was an impossible and unsolvable dilemma. My life or hers? I began doing death maths in my head; how, when, how long, the probability of all the risks and factors. Repeat. Worry. Sadness. Fear. Calculate. Recalculate. Anxiety. The first few moments of waking each day would be clear and calm and then these unwelcome thoughts and feelings would arrive en masse to fill my mind and my day.

Appointments were quickly made. Things began moving at speed. I met my oncologist on the afternoon of Thursday 21st August. If cancer is the villain of this story, then he is the hero – in fact, superhero. He is attractive, compassionate, knowledgeable, intelligent and direct. I could go on, but I won't… actually, I will; he wears cool suits and speaks dulcet Antipodean tones and has a penchant for Green and Black's chocolate. I developed a major teenage-type crush on my oncologist the moment I clapped eyes on him. My major teenage crush has not faded over the years. He is quite simply awesome and gorgeous and utterly fantastic, my lifeboat in the sea of devastation and destruction. I will never forget or stop appreciating the care and kindness he gave me then and in the years to follow.

> *When there is so much uncertainty and unknown we look for a safe and secure base, someone that we can trust and who will be there for us, and my oncologist became that person for me. I felt at 'stage 1' (page 317) with his care, experience, knowledge and reassurance, but the attachment was 'insecure' (page 317) because he was not constantly or consistently available. This created anxiety and fear when I could not be reassured by him.*

I had seen an obstetrician in the morning at a different hospital and got the feeling that no one quite knew what to do with me. I felt buffeted around from hospital to hospital, consultant to consultant. Cancer and pregnancy – there's a dilemma, there's a talking point, there's a medical learning opportunity. There's a fucking great problem. A fucking great problem I was having to go through, one uncomfortable conversation at a time. As far as I could work out, there were three options: do nothing until the baby was born and risk my longer-term survival; have an early baby with the risks and issues that come with a premature baby; or start chemo and take the associated risks for both of us. The obstetrician suggested that an early baby at thirty weeks would present a different set of issues both in the short and long term.

The oncologist was recommending beginning chemotherapy immediately (chemotherapy, or chemo, is a systemic treatment and works by interrupting how cells divide – it can be given in different ways depending on the type of cancer. The chemotherapy can affect other quickly dividing cells causing side effects to cells in the hair, blood cells and lining of the mouth), like that afternoon, as there was a 6cm by 5cm tumour in my breast and a 4cm by 4cm tumour in my armpit. That'll be another big fat FUCK. My ignorance of what this meant to my chances of survival helped me get through the hours to come. The chemo would be followed by surgery, radiotherapy and possibly ongoing hormone treatment. This was going to take longer than I first thought.

Thankfully both doctors had clinics at the same hospital on Thursdays and met at lunchtime to arrange a care plan that would give the best chance of both of us surviving. I would have two cycles of chemo to hold the tumours at bay and then have four weeks off to recover, before a planned Caesarean mid-October (ten days before her due date). So I wouldn't be needing the second natural and drug-free birth plan either. The third cycle of chemo would take place a week after her birth, followed by cycles four, five and six at three-weekly intervals, which would take me to the end of the year. That was the plan. I began to process what the obstetrician and oncologist had told me, but I was reluctant to receive any treatment until I knew exactly what I was dealing with. Even though the fine needle biopsy had diagnosed cancer, I wanted to know exactly what type of cancer it was. Somewhere in my mind was the hope that this was all a horrible mistake.

My 'be perfect' driver (page 329) was challenged and I felt a failure for having cancer. I was relying on my 'try harder' driver (page 329) to sort this out and work through my thoughts and feelings. I used my 'be strong' driver (page 329) to prevent me from breaking down emotionally during the appointments with the obstetrician and oncologist.

I was learning fast that being treated for, and living with, cancer seems to be a series of difficult conversations, choices and consequences. These are punctuated with lots of waiting and unknowns, all of which take a toll physically and emotionally.

The oncologist agreed to a delay of two weeks while a further biopsy was taken and analysed, which allowed a window of time to get used to the idea of what lay ahead. Hell was what lay ahead, sometimes it went beyond hell.

I was avoiding the 'freedom' (page 322) of making a choice about the treatment for as long as possible because I wanted to avoid the responsibility and consequences of my choice. Part of me was still in the 'denial' (page 326) stage of grief. I still held onto hope that the biopsy would show that I didn't have cancer and so I wouldn't have to face the diagnosis of cancer and make a choice about treatment. I used this time to try and gain 'acceptance' (page 327) of what was going to happen and feel 'in control' (page 333) when so much felt 'out of control' (page 333). Asking for a delay to the start of chemo contradicted my 'please others' driver (page 330) because I was usually a good and compliant patient. This left me feeling scared and anxious that if I didn't do what was suggested I was putting myself at risk.

The core biopsy (where samples are taken from several parts of the tumour and are sent for a more in-depth analysis than the fine needle biopsy) was arranged. The difference between the equipment to take a fine needle biopsy and a core biopsy is, in reality, a few millimetres, at the most, but on my breast it felt like several metres.

A local anaesthetic was given to my breast around the tumour. An ultrasound was then used to guide a needle into the tumour and take samples; it sounded like a cap gun being fired. The cap gun was fired about ten times into different parts of the tumour. I squirmed as it took place and felt faint afterwards. I sat outside the room, on the grey plastic chairs, crying and wondering what was happening to my life and how I'd got to this point and so quickly. Out of all the investigations and treatments I have had, this remains the worst. My breast was sore, swollen, bleeding and bruised.

The next appointment on my treatment tour was to have the tumour outlined with a tattoo so that when it came time for the surgery element, the surgeon would know where the original site of the tumour was. As it turned out it was tattoos. There were no pretty flowers, beautiful birds or elaborate initials in a palate of pastel shades. These were large, round, black tattoos which resembled something like a fairy ring around the tumour. Goodbye beautiful, flawless, silky smooth breasts. Cancer and my life as a cancer patient were becoming more visible by the hour.

We returned for the core biopsy results a week later. I sat, hugely pregnant, feeling helpless and surrounded by an ocean of shit. The results had been counted and verified. I had a rare invasive lobular cancer which was grade 1 (the least aggressive type of cancer). The cancer was strongly dependant on oestrogen and unaffected by progesterone, which meant that I would receive ongoing treatment in tablet form once the chemo had ended.

Now I had to decide what the fuck I was going to do. I could avoid my choice no longer, the results were back and now I had to choose. How could I choose between myself and my baby? Loving mum or heartless bitch? I couldn't – I was so overwhelmed with the magnitude of my choice. In the end, Ian said to start the chemo and in a microsecond my decision was made; I just needed someone to tell me what to do. At the time there had not been much research into the long-term effects of chemotherapy on unborn babies, but the oncologist had said he had successfully treated another lady and that was good enough for me. I trusted what he said and it felt good; a relief to get started with the treatment. He would sort this out for me; he was clever and knowledgeable.

I experienced a great deal of anxiety around my 'freedom' (page 322) of choice about what treatment to take and when. It was extremely difficult to choose as there were lots of risks and unknowns with each choice. I felt I had failed at my 'configurations of self' (page 332) of being a good mum because I had failed to keep my baby safe when that was a major part of the role. I was now putting her at risk by choosing to have the chemo while I was pregnant with her and save my life. It was an unsolvable dilemma.

I signed the consent form (consent forms are required for each stage of treatment and give the patient's permission for the treatment to take place. The doctor explains the reason for the treatment and the potential risks and side effects) and hoped for the best. This seemed like the least awful of the available choices, rather than the right or best choice. I felt deeply guilty and traumatised about potentially killing my baby in what, at the time, felt like a selfish act of saving my own life.

Now I knew what the treatment plan was, I launched straight into a practical approach as a coping strategy, trying to gain some control of what was going to be happening. I planned childcare for the lovely Poppy, who was already becoming traumatised by the changes in routine and being left with family while I attended endless hospital appointments. She wasn't old enough to understand any of it, which was as much a blessing as it was a curse. We were all suffering with the change in routine and unpredictability, and the treatment and the physical side effects hadn't even started yet.

I felt like a lost child not knowing who, where or what was going to be able to help me. The world had become a very frightening and unsafe place. To cope with the powerful emotional 'trauma' (page 332) and anxiety, I became very 'logical' (page 332), practical and detached, to counterbalance these intense and uncomfortable feelings, in an attempt to feel stable

and safe again as well as to protect myself emotionally
from the reality of my situation.

There were many appointments over the next few days, in several different locations, to prepare myself and baby for the treatment; treatment for cancer, treatment for cancer while I was pregnant. As a competent multitasker it was proving difficult to hold myself together in appointments and take in the volumes of information I was being given, so I just sat there in a daze, frozen, surviving moment by moment. There were steroid injections to improve her lungs in case the treatment triggered labour and she arrived early. The injections were emotionally bearable as they were going to help her.

Then came a tour of the chemo suite, a tour that no one wants to make. A tour where I completely broke down, sobbing uncontrollably with the prospect of what was going to happen, big heaving sobs that I could neither control nor cease. This was now frighteningly real. This was about to be my reality, a reality of unknowns and uncertainty. I was meeting the staff, seeing the room, the tables, the chairs where I was going to receive my potentially, and hopefully, life-saving treatment which may kill or harm my baby. There are no words, condolences or polite but pointless platitudes for that. This was life at the raw, shit and painful end of the spectrum.

It was at this point the 'denial' (page 326), 'logical' (page 332) and 'be strong' driver (page 329) strategies failed. I was broken emotionally and traumatised by the reality of what was about to happen. I had

no coping strategy to manage my intense thoughts,
feelings, fear and sadness or the possible consequences
from the 'freedom' (page 322) of my choice.

I left the chemo suite with a big white bag of medicines which had unfamiliar names, and I felt resentful and angry at having to take them and risk damaging my baby, my beautiful, innocent baby who I was already in love with and fiercely protective about. It went against my intuitive, unconscious desire and instinct to protect my baby from harm. It went against my values, ethics, morals and principles as a mother. It went against every cell in my mind, soul and body. FUCK YOU CANCER. How dare you put me in this hideous position where I have to choose between two lives. My survival instinct and instinct as a mother to protect were at war, constantly raging in my head. How dare you take away the happiness and love and conversations and plans of growing an innocent person in my belly, and replace it with choices that no one wants to make and medicines that no one wants to take. Every kick and movement was a precious and reassuring sign that things in my belly were okay. I lived for those kicks.

I was starting to feel 'angry' (page 326) at what
cancer was taking from me and how it was changing
the 'meaning' (page 322) of my life.

CHAPTER 3

"My heart is, and always will be, yours."

Jane Austen

The first chemo took place on 1st September 2003. Who knew what the day would hold, who would still be alive at the end of it, but I had no choice, I had to go. The day began with steroids. Every tablet I took felt like I was poisoning myself and my baby. Each tablet was laden with guilt at what I was doing and yet it was crucial for the chemo to take place. Poppy was dropped at a crèche, which we had hastily arranged and hoped would give her some continuity and stability while I was having my treatment. I walked away smiling and waving at her as calmly as I could and we set off for the hospital, but I wanted to scream and shout at the injustice of it all. We arrived at the chemo suite an hour later, my heart heavy with sadness and guilt, my gorgeous, precious and bulging thirty-two-week-pregnant

27

belly protruding into the early autumn sunshine. My hand was on my belly constantly, checking things were still okay in there.

I passed the checking-in challenge. My details matched their details, so I could proceed for the cold cap (the cold cap chills the hair follicles on your head and prevents them from being damaged by the chemo and can stop the hair loss) to be fitted. I decided to wear the cold cap in an attempt to stop my hair falling out. However hopeless it all felt, I at least had to try. The cap was like a very thick swimming hat and was tightly secured with several straps. It's far from a good look and it's far from a comfortable feel. Ian whispered that I resembled a vivisection monkey. Thanks. The cap was then connected to a variety of tubes, which in turn were connected to a machine that looks similar to an air conditioning unit. The machine was turned on and gradually I felt a chill creeping through me, and there I remained for several hours. The cold cap is more of a freezing cap, so the name is a tad misleading.

My 'self-actualisation' (page 331) was trying to focus on something I could do and feel 'in control' (page 333) of, to stabilise the chaos in my life and mind. Focusing on trying to prevent hair loss distracted me from the thoughts and feelings about what I was doing and the risks I was taking having the chemo while I was pregnant.

After forty-five minutes of head freezing, I was wrapped in several blankets, and despite the heat of the day I was so cold I was shivering. The first drug, Adriamycin, was administered; a bright-red drug which alarmingly turned my pee the same shade. Next in was Cytoxan, along with anti-sickness medication and more wearing of the cold cap. In the world of oncology this treatment combination is known as 'AC'.

Pleasant time-filling chat took place amongst the other patients receiving their life-extending drugs on that sunny autumn afternoon. We shared and listened to snippets of each other's lives; how we had all arrived in that chemo suite on that afternoon. Even though I was surrounded by people, I felt extremely isolated and was still wondering how the fuck this was happening to me. I went home a couple of hours later not knowing what to expect and fearful that the kicks would stop. Those kicks kept my heart beating and my hope alive; if they stopped I didn't know how I would cope.

Over the next few days I began to feel tired, and then really tired, as the fast-growing cells in my body (hair, blood and mouth lining) began to die away, hopefully taking a few of those bastard cancer cells out with them. I lived day-by-day, minute-by-minute and kick-by-kick.

Poppy began to develop separation anxiety as our timetable of toddler events was replaced by her being cared for by unfamiliar people in unfamiliar settings. It was hard to watch her tears and distress as she was handed over yet again. I felt a total bitch. Through spending consistent quality time with her once the treatment had ended, her anxiety lessened and she returned to a secure attachment but it was tough going for us both. There was a schedule of appointments for both me and the baby, which were exhausting. It felt like a full-time job commuting between consultants, counties and hospitals.

Two weeks passed and I returned to hospital for a check-up. Another doctor in another room reported I had had a good response to the first cycle of chemo, with the breast tumour shrinking to 4cm by 4cm and the armpit tumour to 2cm by 2cm. His words soothed the angst in my head. Momentarily, relief and hope were savoured.

Towards the end of September, my lovely brother was getting married in France to his French fiancée. I *so* wanted to attend, but only if it was safe for me to do so and, more importantly, safe for the baby. My determined 'fuck you' side said yes, but my maternal instinct guided me to proceed with caution. It was these pockets of potential joy that kept me going on through something so traumatic, with something to aim for, enjoy and achieve; my first of many 'fuck you cancer' moments. A prenatal check declared the thirty-five-week baby and I were doing well and we had the okay to go. It was with great excitement and high-speed packing that we set off for France on a warm and sunny day, with our hair blowing in the wind on the ferry deck. We ate chips and watched England, cancer and chemo fade into the horizon. Gulls were trying keep up in the blue sky above us as if escorting us. Poppy was chatting and giggling away; moments of happiness, moments of my life as it used to be and all that I loved, moments of how it should have been. It felt normal. I felt normal. Normal felt a lifetime ago.

During this trip I could avoid what my life had become and being defined by cancer. I was free to be myself. I could be free from the 'trauma' (page 332), the sadness, the fear and the fighting against the 'configuration of self' (page 332) as a cancer patient.

A few hundred miles and a couple of baguettes later we arrived at a gorgeous hotel with my family waiting. We had just about taken over the whole hotel and the atmosphere was fun and exciting. This was more me. It was a very special weekend, with the French and English guests enjoying separate dinners the night before the wedding. The church wedding was eclectic with touches of English and French culture and tradition woven throughout. Vows were exchanged in both languages. A big red double-decker London bus transported us from the church to the reception, looking both magnificent and out of place in the green landscape of the French countryside.

The wedding reception was held in the ruins of a monastery. As dusk overtook day, the ruins were lit by torches of fire, creating mesmerising and ever-changing shadows on the stone walls as a gentle breeze fanned them. The setting was stunning and the food superb, an abundance of history and architecture bombarding our senses; photo line-ups, chic French couture, laughter, smiling faces, emotional speeches, table dancing, a traditional French wedding cake which looked about forty feet tall and a chance to catch up with friends and family. Cancer was nowhere to be seen or heard; a brief interlude from the shitness that had gone before and which still lay ahead. We rolled, exhausted, to bed in the early hours.

After another delicious carb-laden breakfast we met again for lunch, sitting outside at long tables cloaked in crisp white linen, under the shady branches of an enormous tree. We enjoyed more courses and conversations, but time was ticking away from fun and happiness and towards goodbyes, drugs and chemo. The tears began to well and then trickle and then fall and, for the second time, they were falling uncontrollably. I was unable to say goodbye as I was too overwhelmed with emotion. With heaving sobs, reluctance and fear I got back in the car to drive away from all that I loved and enjoyed.

We unpacked from our France trip and I began taking the steroids in preparation for chemo number two, which was equally worrying and every bit as traumatic as number one. I had become very attached to and protective over my baby and clung to the hope she would survive until birth and be healthy, should we get that far. Every pill and every droplet of chemo was me taking a risk of that not happening. She had become my focus, my obsession, my hope, my world, my *raison d'être,* which distracted and protected me from thinking about the seriousness of the situation. The guilt of the risks I was taking was difficult to manage. Life and death hung precariously for us both. We were going through this experience together, inseparable and bonded. She was my reason to keep going. I had constant feelings that I had failed her as a mother. I had failed to provide her with a safe, nurturing space from which to enter this world. The anxiety and trauma were immense.

I was in the midst of repeated 'trauma' (page 332) and had nowhere that felt safe and secure. There was neither the time nor space to process or recover from one trauma before the next one arrived and my mental health was being gradually eroded with each trauma.

The hair loss started virtually to the day and hour the pastel-coloured leaflet said it would. I went to the loo at 6pm, and my pubic hair was intact. I went again at 10pm, just four short hours later, and all my pubic hair was detached, lying there in my big pregnancy pants like a dead rodent. Bit by bit my hair, my femininity, my identity was falling out, abandoning me. I wanted to abandon me and pop back when it was all sorted and back to normal. Over the coming days my brunette hair made it everywhere, like a Hansel and Gretel trail, on pillows, floors and work surfaces. The final straw was finding my hair in the freezer; I hadn't even gone to the freezer.

Not knowing if my hair was going to totally fall out was stressful and another unknown. I went to my hairdressers and had it shaved off to a short crew cut; it was unfeminine and unflattering and I was charged £20 for the privilege, but I was in control. I tried to make myself look funky, as if it was part of my conscious identity, a lifestyle choice rather than medically induced. It worked to a degree but inside it was far from the truth. I was a cauldron crew-cutted pregnant woman of sadness, fear and anger.

The hair loss was out of my 'control' (page 333) and was creating anxiety in the process, by the unknown of whether it was or wasn't going to fall out. By having it cut off I felt 'in control' (page 333), although I didn't like the consequence of the 'freedom' (page 322) of my choice and how I now looked. I wanted the hairdresser to see me as a 'victim' (page 328) and not charge me for the annihilation of my locks and in turn the impact on my looks and femininity.

Chemo number two followed the same routine as number one but my emotions were more intense. Each time the risks increased. I had got away without harming her the first time round. Would I be so lucky this time? More drugs, more risks, more anxiety.

I then had a four-week break from chemo to recover and to prepare for the birth. Just get her out safely. Just let me see her, touch her, smell her, hear her, wrap her up and protect her from any other risk ever again. This time was tainted by the unknown and uncertainty. It was always there, just hovering, never quite leaving. The kicks and antenatal appointments kept coming. I wrote a will and planned my funeral, just in case. I sobbed through both. Writing a will is hard enough when we are healthy; it goes against our survival instinct to write about our death; when you are losing your hair and at times your mind, and you are pregnant and mid-cycles of cancer treatment, it is harder. We may have needed this for real, so it was a serious and sombre affair and felt important to get right.

Finally, the day of her birth was here – Tuesday 14th October 2003 – thirty-eight weeks into a pregnancy which had started off so perfectly. One diagnosis of cancer, two cycles of chemo and countless uncomfortable conversations later, somehow we had made it to this day. We rose early and travelled to the hospital in darkness and silence, both scared to speak or be hopeful. We arrived at the ward at sunrise; this felt auspicious. The questions from the nursing staff quickly began. A delay swiftly followed because the obstetric team was not aware of my cancer treatment. I began to fight holding back the tears. I just wanted her out and safe, to know she was okay. The waiting began. Blood was taken and I waited for it be analysed to ensure it would be safe to operate. It was upsetting and tiring to explain my situation to each team and each shift change. Just say hello, read the fucking notes. Do what you've got to do and leave.

My resilience had been worn down and I was becoming less and less tolerant of minor inconveniences.

The obstetrician who had monitored me throughout the pregnancy had booked a Caesarean for the day that he was at the hospital so he could be there. He stroked my crew-cutted head softly and rhythmically as I was prepped for her birth. I tried to enjoy the moment. I'd had a Caesarean with Poppy so was aware of the procedure which was to follow. The epidural was unpleasant but necessary. I felt compelled to explain to all present that I was pubeless through cancer treatment not lifestyle choice; we all giggled. That was the last time I remember giggling for a while. Cold surged into my spine. Soon after, sensation left my legs. A catheter was inserted and I was manoeuvred around the bed and quiet began to fall in the room. Instruments clunked behind a screen improvised from a sheet. My head was still being stroked. It felt comforting and reassuring.

A paediatric team was also present, along with the obstetric and anaesthetic team on standby, as no one really knew what was going to happen. The room was crowded. Bystanders. Gladiators, ready to deliver, protect and, if necessary, save. This was it, the moment I had hoped for, but also not dared hope for. The room felt tense. I could feel rummaging and pulling in my belly. At 12.11 she was born. She was silent; there was now rushing about behind the improvised sheet screen, and then a noise, the noise of a crying baby. I, of course, instantly started to cry. I couldn't see, I couldn't touch, I couldn't smell, I couldn't move, but I could hear. I could hear her proclaiming her arrival into the world, away from the drugs and death my body contained.

After what seemed an eternity she was passed to me, tightly wrapped. She was gorgeous, and with considerably more hair than me and I, cried again. Delight and relief could be felt in the parts I could feel. She was here, she was breathing, she was alive and she was instantly the most precious thing I had ever seen, touched, smelt, heard or hoped for.

How do you name a baby that has meant so much, been through so much and become your reason to keep going when you didn't think you could? We decided on Bonnie Scarlett. Bonnie was born ten days early weighing 8lbs 3oz. Bonnie needed a blood test just to check she was healthy, which she was. We began telling our friends and family that Bonnie was here. Bonnie was alive and Bonnie appeared healthy. Bonnie, Bonnie, Bonnie. My world now began each sentence with her name. My heart filled with love and protection for her. No, I didn't want Bonnie to be looked after on the first night of her life; I had waited a nervous and anxious two months to meet her and I didn't want her to leave my side. I slept with my hand on the cot next to me.

The build-up and focus of her birth, and the high following it, was swiftly replaced with a deep and vast depression and the enormity of months of treatment and uncertainty which lay ahead of me. Tears permanently filled my eyes. I looked round the ward to the happy smiling faces of families, doting on and bonding with their babies. I was upset that this wasn't what I was enjoying; my fundamental right as a mother. Hearts and faces full of love and hope. I was facing months of treatment, shitness and uncertainty. A desperate phone call to the lovely breast care nurse was made and she came to the rescue. Although no one could take away my fear and pain, she was a kind, safe and knowledgeable base, and grounded me in the chaos of my mind. How was I going to cope with months of treatment, a new baby, a toddler, a Caesarean section and a head full of hopelessness? The tears flowed and the anxiety and anger rumbled away inside me.

The focus and hope I had placed on Bonnie formed part of my protective 'denial' (page 326) of what was happening to me. Once she was safely born, this left me to face the 'loss' (page 325) and the impact cancer was having on me. The coping strategies of 'denial' (page 326) and my 'be strong' driver (page 329) were unable to suppress my feelings and I experienced a deep 'depression' (page 326) and hopelessness. Cancer fast-tracked me back to 'stage 1' (page 317) where I was seeking comfort and safety from someone because my existence was under threat. However, as adults, there is an unsolvable conflict: we are unable to be soothed in the same way as a young child because we are aware of 'death' (page 321); ultimately no one can save us from this.

We came home from hospital with Bonnie to flowers, cards and an answerphone full of messages; word had quickly spread. Poppy thought it was just great to have a new toy to play with, a real live doll. At sixteen months old she didn't share the same sense of protection, relief or understanding. She was an innocent bystander of the carnage that my life and our lives had become. I became a guard, always checking where they both were; safe, checking. Checking, checking, checking. I pinned on big beaming smiles for visitors and at medical appointments to hide my sadness, desolation, vulnerability, isolation, anxiety and fear.

CHAPTER 4

"The thing about perspective-changing events
is that they usually don't announce themselves as such."

Andrea Goeglein

We were soon back in hospital for pre-chemo checks; another doctor in another room. Chemo cycle number three was just around the corner. No time to treasure the first few days of a precious baby. The cancer timetable supersedes all else, marching on. Bonnie made her debut in the oncology clinic to 'ooohs' and 'ahhhhs'. But the focus then swiftly shifted to the obligatory physical examination which would gauge what had happened and would determine what would happen next. The examination revealed that the cancer had had no response to chemo round two. It remained static, nothing had changed. The anxiety and anger continued to grow and gnaw away inside me. I felt as if I hadn't tried hard enough.

I had again made naïve assumptions. I expected chemo to be like taking paracetamol or antibiotics; that it would just work. I was beginning to learn that cancer is like no other illness, and there is no predictable pathway or guaranteed treatment outcome. It was agreed that I would have one more cycle of the AC drug combination.

The routine and utter exhaustion of a new baby and a toddler were all-consuming. Ian is a night owl by nature and took on the night feed duties. We discussed employing a temporary night nurse but spent the money on employing a cleaner instead, subconsciously hoping they would be able to clear up the mess surrounding us; the trail of carnage that cancer was leaving in its wake, and all that cancer was stealing and changing.

There was no breastfeeding option. The milk would be tainted with chemo and would be a poison for Bonnie instead of nutritional and nourishing. I suspected that additional hormones wouldn't be good for me either, so I was given medication to stop the milk production. My boobs swelled and swelled, gorged with poisoned milk, until the medication did what it was supposed to do and they receded. The formula milk we had chosen for Bonnie was too rich and she was frequently puking up bottles of the stuff at 3am, which then required bedding and clothing changes and then refeeding. A volume of washing was generated. Additional linen was purchased. Life was tiring, stressful and now smelt of milky vomit.

I presented for the third round of chemo when Bonnie was just a week old. It was heartbreaking to arrive at the chemo suite with an innocent and precious baby who had already been through so much before she was born. She didn't deserve this; she should have been in a nice warm buggy enjoying the colours and chill of autumn. The process began again. She was cooed over. I just wanted to get on with the treatment. At least I didn't have to think about the damage the chemo was potentially causing Bonnie now. The damage was all mine, my consequence; I was on my own now, she was out, she was safe and I was now travelling solo and lonely on my journey of hell. Her face and tiny body both comforted me and pained me. I wanted to be there for her and the thought of the treatment not working and having to say goodbye was unbearable.

Although I had very deep protective feelings for Bonnie, I found it difficult to fully bond with her because I was unsure that I would live long enough to see her first Christmas or birthday, let alone the childhood milestones and the rites of passage into teenage and adult life. The tussles in my head continued. Why would I bond and have the pain of having to say goodbye? Not bonding and keeping safe seemed easier and yet so sad. It was a defensive position of self-preservation and yet part of me craved to open my heart and let the love flow and to take the risk. The thought of dying and leaving two young children with no recollection or a sense of who I was deepened my depression.

I continued to experience 'trauma' (page 332) from each piece of news that didn't give me hope I was going to live. My fear of dying and the uncertainty of the unknown were eroding my mental health on a daily basis. My 'configuration of self' (page 332) about being a good mother was further challenged when I found it difficult to bond with Bonnie.

The side effects of the third cycle of chemo were similar to one and two. Tiredness followed by fatigue and a mouth so full of ulcers I couldn't talk or eat, and then brighter and better but tainted because I began counting down the days until it all began again. Just as my mind was being battered emotionally, so was my body, physically. I was frequenting the doctor's with bouts of sinusitis after each chemo cycle. Antibiotics were prescribed, administered, taken and re-requested. It felt like my life and body were failing me. I was unbelievably angry. The list was growing of things I was angry about; dark, grey days of winter, days just to tick off, days just to endure. I thought making it to the chemo halfway point would lighten my mood, but it didn't; it just got worse.

I was constantly letting go of the 'social dimension' (page 323) and 'personal dimension' (page 324) of my life as well as my hopes and plans. I realised my life lacked fulfilment in my 'spiritual' (page 324) dimension too and I was experiencing increasing 'isolation' (page 322) and 'depression' (page 326) in the process. I was just physically surviving and so my life had less and less 'meaning' (page 322) and the cycle of feeling more hopeless, depressed and angry continued. The 'unfinished business' (page 331) of not knowing whether the treatment would work, whether I would live or die, was constantly causing me anxiety.

The pre-treatment check, ahead of the fourth cycle of chemo, identified I had had no response to the previous two chemo cycles and the registrar needed to check with the oncologist about what to do. We left the hospital not knowing what would follow. It felt liberating to be free from the treatment timetable but also frightening not to know what would be next.

Although Ian and I had been together for four years, we had never got round to getting married as it hadn't seemed important. Cancer changed that. We wanted to tidy things up and make our relationship more formal and so we discussed marriage. It seemed a welcome distraction to the destruction, and now Bonnie was here safe and well, it was something else that was positive to think about.

Ian had taken the day off work and we were choosing an engagement ring in the Lanes shopping area of Brighton when the call came through from the registrar. I stepped outside of the shop into the bustling street to take the call. I was told I would be switching to a drug called docetaxel, which also meant switching to another hospital to have it administered. My stomach lurched. Not the conversation you want to be having when you are choosing diamond cuts and ring sizes, but life as a cancer patient goes on. The dose of steroids for this drug was different and the registrar stressed the importance of taking these correctly. It was all change. It was all unsettling. It all continued to be fucking awful.

Cancer involves a lot of waiting and not knowing; neither of which I am so good with. I like to know and get on, to be proactive, to take an action, to do something, to try, anything. Now I had to get used to a new routine and let go of the predictability of the last. My head was spinning with the practicalities. The pre-chemo checks were done on the same day as treatment, which meant a longer day at the hospital but only one hospital trip. Food, childcare, Ian's birthday and business all buzzed through my brain at speed, like a quiz show question which I had thirty seconds to answer.

Happy fortieth birthday to Ian. Happy fourth chemo to me. What a way to spend your fortieth birthday, taking your wife and one-month-old baby to a chemo suite. The steroids were taken. Poppy was dropped off and we journeyed to hospital number three for the next part of the treatment. Ian was really suffering with stress at this time and was finding it hard to cope. He was worried about me, the children, our future (if there was going to be one) and his business. He dropped me at the hospital with Bonnie and stayed outside to make work phone calls. I ventured in to state my name and begin the process again; new building, new people, new conversations about diagnosis and treatment regimes. I had to sign that I had taken the steroids before the chemo would be administered. This must be serious. The cold cap was fitted and off we went again, with Bonnie sleeping in her buggy while life and death, treatment and hope, surrounded her. One of my saddest moments was watching the chemo going into one arm and holding Bonnie while I fed her in the other, the polarities of life within my arms. Eight hours later we left.

We met up with Ian's friends in the evening for a birthday meal. I was woozy with the drugs but put on my smiley 'I'm-just-fine' face. I could not wait to get home and take it off.

The 'be strong' driver (page 329), 'logical' (page 332) and 'in control' (page 333) strategies were failing no matter how hard I tried to maintain them. I was lonely, isolated, vulnerable, scared and angry. The repeated 'trauma' (page 332), with no hope or guarantee of the outcome, was draining me. I was fighting against the new 'configuration of self' (page 332) of being a cancer patient, and I wanted to go back to the 'meaning' (page 322) which I had chosen and created for my life, and not have a head full of anger, fear and excruciating sadness.

I experienced several physical side effects with the AC chemo and so it was a bit of a shock when the side effects of the docetaxel started because these were more psychological. I was now suffering from unrelenting and undiminishing anxiety. I was craving calmness and predictability. I knew how the tiredness and mouth ulcers of the AC worked. I didn't know what to do with permanent anxiety and was prescribed lorazepam, which took the edge off things. I handed back the unused tablets at the end of the chemo as I could see how easy it would be to keep taking them. Over the coming months I sometimes regretted that action as they would have soothed and calmed my addled brain very nicely.

It was now mid-winter and the dark, grey days became overwhelming. I couldn't cope with the thought of a whole day, it was too much, too many hours of hideousness to think about. A deep, dark depression took hold. I felt isolated from the life I loved. I felt hopeless and could see no way out. The depression was interspersed with bouts of rage when the tiniest thing went wrong, and anxiety and fear about dying. I could not continue to live like this and began to break the day into two-hour slots and would not let myself think past the two-hour slot I was in. The days became more manageable. I found walking a good distraction, so aimed to walk for half an hour round the village each day. This proved to be a good focus and started a habit of exercising and being outdoors which continues to this day. It felt good exercising out the anger and stress; rhythmical and mobile, being outside with nature and the changing weather, clouds and seasons; trees and leaves, colours and noise; beautiful external distractions from my internal turmoil.

> *My 'self-actualisation' (page 331) found a small way to drive me forward. Taking part in activities which I enjoyed and felt 'in control' (page 333) of created a distraction from my psychological and emotional distress.*

The fifth cycle of chemo and the second dose of docetaxel followed the same pattern as cycle number four. The tumour felt softer; a faint flicker of hope. December 17th began routinely, as with the other days of that winter, with feelings of despair and anxiety. I had taken the girls to the mother and toddler group Christmas party in the morning, where I sat feeling out of place and self-conscious in the room of laughter and festive excitement. In the afternoon we sat drinking tea and eating cake, celebrating Ian's mum's seventieth birthday. Quite suddenly and quickly I began to feel unwell. I had to carry a card with me which stated that

I was receiving chemo and the steps to take if I felt unwell. I took my temperature and it was 38.5 degrees, which for a chemo patient is dangerous, so I called the hospital.

I was told to come in immediately. Plans were dropped, plans were made; Poppy was cared for by a neighbour and Bonnie came along, still in her Santa babygro. It was the standard hospital start; I gave my name, address, date of birth and chemo card, and the process of waiting and working out what was wrong began. I had no definitive symptoms so the diagnostic process began with a blood test.

Sometime in the early hours of the morning I was diagnosed with neutropenic sepsis. My white blood cell count was dangerously low and I was at risk of dying because I had no means of fighting infection. I was now so traumatised I just lay there passive while the new plan was explained. I didn't actually care. Just do what you need to do. The new plan involved being admitted to hospital and having lots of antibiotics. It must be bad as there was no mention of the cancer.

I said my goodbyes to Bonnie and Ian and got in a wheelchair to make the journey to the ward. I had no idea where I was going. I was delivered to an isolation room somewhere in the hospital. I felt too ill and too tired to care. Sleep engulfed my still body. Morning arrived a few hours later and the weak winter light entered the room. There were new rules here. Salad, flowers and visitors were contraband.

My eyes brightened when my oncologist visited a few hours later. I was to remain isolated until my white blood cell count had risen. No one knew how long this would take, maybe a couple of weeks. I'd like to be home for Christmas I thought, but felt too exhausted to say. I lay in bed motionless and dozed through TV programmes, blood tests and intravenous (IV) changes. I had nothing left to give. The sleep was deep and peaceful and my mind welcomed the rest. The antibiotics kept coming, as did the blood tests to monitor their effect. I was happily surprised when the blood count had risen enough two days later to be cautiously discharged, in time for Christmas, with a strict protocol if I felt ill again. I was excited to be set free from my isolation room. I focused my anxiety not on what had happened to me, not on how serious this was, but on how I was going to finish Christmas shopping if I wasn't allowed out to mix with crowds. My mind was protecting me once more.

I had now experienced so much 'trauma' (page 332) that I was unable to detect and register any new trauma and so didn't engage with how serious the hospitalisation had been. Each trauma wiped my sense of connection, hope and achievement away, and so in the end I gave up trying to connect because it all felt so hopeless.

I had lived long enough to see Bonnie's first Christmas, something of a milestone. I felt fragile and withdrawn, devoid and disconnected from life. I thought back to a year ago, Poppy's first Christmas, a happy affair of excitement. Now a year, a cancer diagnosis and a baby later, this; a day I wanted to be a part of and yet was terrified cancer would take me away from. I found it hard to join in and be happy.

By the time I got to chemo cycle number six at the end of December 2003, I was exhausted. I was exhausted with the stress, I was exhausted with the treatment, I was exhausted with the unknown, I was exhausted with the uncertainty, I was exhausted with the prospect of several more months of treatment ahead of me, I was exhausted with having a nineteen-month-old child and a two-month-old child to care for and a husband who was finding it hard to hold it all together. I went home to see in the New Year – a broken woman, barely able to lift my head off the sofa as I felt so drained physically and emotionally.

I had nothing consistently safe or stable in my life and this, along with the constant uncertainty, had a detrimental impact on my psychological and emotional health. I was worn down by the relentless 'trauma' (page 332) of being a cancer patient and not feeling I had any support or strategies to cope with my feelings.

CHAPTER 5

*"Your present circumstances don't determine where you can go;
they merely determine where you start."*

Nido Qubein

The post-chemo check-up in early January 2004 revealed that the chemo had finally done its work and there were no 'palpable lumps', which was a minor miracle considering my starting position. Chemo was done but there is no rest for a cancer patient. I was referred to join another waiting list to meet another consultant and even more rotating registrars.

I had wanted another baby before cancer invaded my life, and was brave enough to ask of the possibility of this during the check-up appointment. It was quietly suggested in a voice devoid of pitch that this would not be a good idea as having the least amount of hormones possible in my body would provide the best chance of survival. I left with tears falling down my cheeks, again; another choice that cancer had taken away from me. I was grieving once more. I would never see the positive blue pregnancy test line again. I would never feel a baby kick inside me again. I would never flick through a baby name book again, lining up initials to check for rude or funny acronyms. I would never coo over tiny babygros again. Fuck you cancer. I wanted to have a pregnancy and birth and a child that was full of happiness and love, not filled with chaos and chemo, fear and depression. It took me a very long year to grieve and accept that I wouldn't have any more children; a very long year of an empty feeling, deep inside me; a very long year of false happiness and congratulations as my friends announced their second and third babies.

> *Not being able to have any more children was a further 'loss' (page 325) and perhaps one of the greatest I faced, and I needed to grieve for this. I was angry at not having the 'freedom' (page 322) to choose to have another baby. I had 'unfinished business' (page 331) at not being able to have a healthy pregnancy and in the desire to relive and repair this by having another child.*

I began taking tamoxifen ten days after finishing my sixth cycle of chemo. Tamoxifen is an anti-oestrogen drug and can be used to treat breast cancer in pre- and post-menopausal women who have oestrogen hormone receptive breast cancer. This type of breast cancer has proteins called receptors, which the hormones attach to, stimulating the cancer cells to divide and grow. Tamoxifen fits onto the receptor and prevents the cancer from growing. My cancer was hormone receptive and required hormones to continue growing. This was good news in that I could take ongoing medicine to reduce the risk of that cancer returning, but bad news in that I wondered how I could reduce my hormone levels. Although I trusted my oncologist implicitly, I did question whether I had all the right treatment and did contemplate seeking a second opinion. But I also wondered where this would end, and recognised that I would keep going until I found the answer I wanted. The answer I wanted would be that the cancer wouldn't come back and I wasn't going to die. No one was ever going to give me that answer and so I stopped.

I was desperately searching for safety and reassurance that I was not going to die and about what I could 'influence' (page 333). I was trying to delete 'death' (page 321) from my life and was searching for someone or something to take that away from me, but no one or anything could because 'death' (page 321) is an 'existential given' (page 321) of life.

My appointment for the surgical referral arrived and would take place back at the first hospital, where it had all started, one pregnancy, two hospitals, five months, one head of hair and two eyebrows ago. I attended the surgery appointment reluctantly, knowing I would see the spectacled surgeon again. I was still angry at him for how he had delivered my diagnosis. I was silent and detached through the examination and explanation of the procedure. I signed the consent form and the surgery was scheduled. Another pastel-shaded leaflet was explained and handed over; what I should be aware of and would need for this tranche of treatment. Pyjamas. I had no pyjamas. I reluctantly went shopping for pyjamas. The shop assistant was marvelling over my purchases and was excited for me about my new pyjamas. I was not excited. If only you knew why I needed these, I thought, fighting to hold back both tears and anger. I wanted to cry and shout and scream. I didn't want pyjamas or surgery, but I would need both if I wanted to live.

Outwardly I was compliantly and passively going along with the cancer treatment, but I was 'angry' (page 326) inside at my 'loss' (page 325), lack of 'freedom' (page 322) and lack of 'control' (page 333) at not being able to choose the 'meaning' (page 322) for my life.

I reluctantly made my way to hospital with the unwanted pyjamas on Sunday 8th February 2004 for the surgery, which was scheduled the next day. I was checked in and shown to a side room that a lovely breast care nurse had arranged so the girls could visit at any time. Another lady from a ward a bit further along asked me why I had my own room. I wanted to scream 'BECAUSE I HAVE FUCKING CANCER AND TWO YOUNG CHILDREN AND LIFE IS FUCKING SHIT SO FUCK OFF', but I didn't. Looking back, this was when I was beginning to run really low on energy, patience and spirit. I was moody. I was resentful. I lay there on my pre-surgery hospital bed, my body passive and yet my mind ragefully willing time to pass, wanting to fast-forward from this existence of unhappiness and misery. I found it hard to find satisfaction, pleasure or joy in anything. I didn't want to have to go through the surgery, the drugs, the recovery or the further impingement that cancer created on my life, my choices and my children. This was the last day of having symmetrical boobs. I grieved the loss of my scar-free body. Tomorrow I would look different. I tried to sleep in these unfamiliar surroundings.

The next morning I was examined by several people keen and fresh from their weekends, there to perform their jobs. I was there to lose part of my body, my femininity, my identity. I lay there topless and exposed. I could see the hideous tattoos where 'X' marked the spot of the tumour to guide the spectacled surgeon and his scalpel. I was then drawn upon like an oversized canvas. The big black marker pen tickled as the thick lines it left behind joined the hideous tattoo marks, the signage to the cancer within me. Time ticked by. I was wheeled down to theatre and left to wait; to wait for the needles and drugs and scars. I was looking forward to being unconscious and having a break from the emotional turmoil.

I woke up with no knowledge of the passage of time. My senses began feeding me information; the recovery room, bright lights, my name being said repeatedly, my chest taking deep breaths of air-conditioned air. I was alive. A massive dressing covered my left breast and protruding from the dressing were three tubes, each leading to a clear pressurised bottle. These were to collect the blood and fluid from around the surgery site. The bottles would have to go everywhere I did, clunking and clinking together, their contents being measured and monitored. I felt relief that the cancer had been removed as if I had been exorcised and it was now contained in a pot somewhere, no longer contaminating me.

The time in hospital was okay. I was lucky as the girls were able to visit outside of visiting times and, although I couldn't do much physically, I could at least see them, touch them and smell them. I appreciated the hospital staff being flexible with this. From my hospital bed I could see my dad bringing the girls in, weaving his way through the Victorian streets that surrounded the hospital. I'm pleased they don't have a recollection of those times. I didn't have the energy or mental capacity to be a good mum. They should have been my focus, but my fear and anger took this. They should have had my love and care, but cancer treatment took this.

I was so consumed trying to survive the 'trauma' (page 332) and lack of hope that I could not concentrate on anything else, and this conflicted with my 'configuration of self' (page 332) of being a good mum and being physically and emotionally available to care for my children.

I wasn't great when people visited me; I wanted to withdraw from the world and be left alone to process and heal from the never-ending torrent of treatment and side effects. I craved silence and peace, stillness, quiet, to be left alone and to have no thoughts. I feigned sleep to the nurse who banged on about her boyfriend problems, because I really didn't give a shit, really I didn't. Not a toss. I'll swap you your boyfriend issues for my cancer, I thought from behind my closed eyelids. I just lay there for hour after hour, day after day, willing for time to pass; willing for health and choice and peace of mind.

I was discharged from hospital on the Friday. I was fragile to say the least. The dressing and tubes had been removed, one tube at a time, when they had done their job and the fluid began to recede, as my body worked hard to heal and repair. The tube removal was uncomfortable and it was unpleasant to feel them being pulled through my body. The lovely breast care nurse urged me to look at the scar. I really didn't want to, but I did. It was fucking massive. Thick and red, eight inches long and shaped like a fish hook, starting high in my arm pit, making its way down and then across my breast and back up again like a wobbly 'j' written by a blindfolded two-year-old. My breasts were now hugely uneven and my confidence further plummeted as I looked at the wound.

There was to be no driving for three weeks. Immobile. Not useful when you live in a village in the middle of nowhere. I was given exercises to do to help gain the movement back in my arm and shoulder, but even now, fourteen years on, I still suffer with pain and stiffness and have never regained full movement, sensation or strength. Wire-free bras were now the way forward. Not exactly sexy.

I just wanted to sleep until it was all over, to wake up at another time in another place, far, far away from this. I was now waiting, waiting to recover, waiting to drive, waiting for the pathology report of the tumour, waiting to see what would happen next. Waiting and not knowing. I left with an outpatient appointment in ten days' time and another pastel-shaded leaflet explaining the recovery from the surgery.

Because I had some of my lymph nodes removed from my armpit to check if the cancer was still there, I was also (and remain) at risk of lymphedema (lymphedema is a chronic condition for which there is no cure, where a swelling develops in body tissue and is caused by damage or disruption to the lymphatic system). I am careful not to injure or damage the arm or skin, and wear thick gloves for gardening and don't carry heavy shopping bags.

By the Sunday I was back at hospital. I had developed an uncomfortable build-up of seroma (a collection of clear body fluid that can be caused by the trauma of surgery) under my armpit. Seroma sounds like a posh Italian dish. It isn't. It felt as though I had a cricket ball wedged in there. I went straight to the ward (as outlined in the pastel-shaded leaflet) where some of the fluid was removed using a comedy-sized needle. There is a fine line between drawing the fluid off to ease the discomfort and causing infection, and further trauma, by doing so. Therefore not all the fluid is removed, just enough so it feels more comfortable. My body needed to work out how to reroute the seroma.

I was back again on the Tuesday for further removal of seroma and unexpectedly saw the spectacled surgeon who had the pathology results. It was a heart-stopping moment as I hadn't expected to see him or have the results. I wasn't prepared for this at all. Maybe I should start expecting the unexpected in this world of oncology. The pathology results were read to me. The good news (because we are wired to find the good even in shit situations) was the pathology report showed I had a mixed cancer of grades 1 and 2 of invasive lobular and invasive ductal carcinoma, and only one lymph node of the four sampled had cancer in it. And the bad news was that the pathology report showed there hadn't been a clear margin (a clear margin is when there are no cancer cells on the outer edge of the removed tumour site) of cancer-free cells around the tumour site.

Not having a clear margin meant I would be at greater risk of a recurrence of cancer and I would have to have further surgery to remove these cells and gain a clear margin. I was rescheduled for surgery on 1st March. I was well and truly fucked off by the prospect of this and the thought of going through the process again, with the lack of independence it created, but I had no choice. I had the seroma drawn off a third time by the lovely breast care nurse. On this occasion it was third time lucky and it didn't return. My body had worked it out; I wished my exhausted brain could do the same.

I used the lower cancer grade as part of the 'bargaining' (page 326) to gain 'acceptance' (page 327) of cancer and I felt more hopeful for a future because of this. I was sad at being disfigured by the surgery and avoided engaging with my feelings about this as there was so much else going on. I was 'angry' (page 326) at still being a cancer patient with its lack of 'freedom' (page 322) and not being able to choose the 'meaning' (page 322) I wanted for my life.

I was back at the hospital again on Sunday 28th February, with my pyjamas, prior to the surgery scheduled for the next day. Good job I hadn't burnt the pyjamas. I sat on my bed, protecting my opportunity for life, my surgery slot. I couldn't leave the bed as someone else might take it. So I sat there, waiting and watching.

The operating day began and people were checked, drawn upon and wheeled away, coming back hours later sleepy, still and silent. As the day passed my anger grew. When would it be my turn? The day ticked on and on. Each time the porters came, I hoped it would be my turn; early morning, mid-morning, late morning, lunchtime, early afternoon, mid-afternoon, late afternoon. I was last on the surgery list that Monday and was not operated on until 5.30pm, by which time I was tired, hungry, irritated and thirsty. That day and that wait changed something in me, and the burning rage that I had lived with, which I didn't know how to let out or let go of or even what it was about, morphed that day into what I can only describe as a type of post-traumatic stress. I was decreasingly unable to function or focus on anything. I had been ground down until there was nothing left. I couldn't take any more.

The previous process of surgery was repeated and I woke up crying and agitated in the recovery room. This time there were no drains, just another large dressing; just another agonising wait for the results; just another three weeks without driving; just another trauma. When the results came through at an outpatient appointment two weeks later, there was now a clear margin. Congratulations, I had successfully passed that test and could move to the next challenge. I was referred to another waiting list, another consultant and another stage of treatment: radiotherapy.

This was the lowest point of the treatment. I was so tired and worn down by the repeated 'trauma' (page 332) and because I didn't have a safe and 'secure attachment' (page 316) with anything, that I couldn't recover from them. To get through the diagnosis and treatment I had remained in a very practical and 'logical' (page 333) place. I used my 'anger' (page 326) and 'denial' (page 326) along with my 'be strong' driver (page 329) and 'be perfect' driver (page 329) as coping mechanisms. These had been good for keeping me functioning on a day-to-day basis because I found it impossible to be vulnerable, say I was struggling or to ask for help or support with the emotional and the psychological impact of cancer. Because I had not addressed the underlying feelings, these were now overwhelming me and the coping mechanisms failing me. My mental health was suffering to such an extent that even making simple choices was beyond me.

At some point I had been given a pastel-coloured leaflet about support groups, which I had shoved unread into my handbag, which was then shoved in the cancer file, which was then shoved in a cupboard. I could cope. I was fine. I could handle this. I was strong. I was Bex. The surgery triggered something in me and I began to recognise that I wasn't coping at all. In fact I was failing epically. Falling apart. I now knew I needed to ask for help.

I searched for the cancer file, a whole file of information documenting my life as a cancer patient. I searched through the consent forms, information sheets and emergency cards. I found the details of the monthly breast cancer support group run from hospital number one. I forced myself along nervously, hoping to be rescued from my misery, that it would be taken away and disposed of by someone else. I wanted the answer and the problem to be solved by someone else. I didn't discover for many years that I had the answer and would have to do the work myself.

Although the work and support offered at the group was invaluable, I felt out of place and awkward. I persevered for a couple of meetings, but I just didn't feel my issues were relevant or that I related to the other people there. This increased my feelings of isolation and depression, instead of soothing them. I had taken a risk asking for help and not got what I needed. Actually I had no idea what I needed as there was now so much wrong in and with my life. Maybe I gave up too soon. Maybe I wasn't ready. Maybe it wasn't what I needed. Back to the cupboard. Back to the cancer file.

At this stage I was too traumatised for the support group and needed to address the underlying 'trauma' (page 332) cancer had created, as well as my 'anger' (page 326) and anxiety. My 'self-actualisation' (page 331) was driving me to address my unhappiness.

There was another pastel-shaded leaflet for a cancer support centre also run from hospital number one. My eyes scanned the text. This felt better; a wide range of complementary therapies, support groups and counselling were available. Counselling, even writing that word gives me a sense of comfort, support and warmth. Cancer, and counselling about cancer, was about to become a catalyst for so much.

It was hard to ask for help, to be vulnerable and say I was failing. I was fun, strong, bold and energetic Bex; always lively, always with a crazy idea and never far from doing something funny or different. But I was trapped in a bottomless, inescapable pit of fear and anger. I could not see a way out or through. How to escape, how to free myself? My strategies were not working and I knew of no others. They were failing in a catastrophic way and in turn so was I. I was slipping away, exhausted, tired of trying. There was a subconscious sense that the support centre would be a safe place and I trusted that sense. I knew I needed support and help to recover from the emotional and psychological side effects of cancer, just as I needed help and time to recover physically from the treatment. But for now I didn't know how. If I couldn't sort this out, who could? I had always been so capable. I had never failed at anything or had to ask for support. I had never been weak or sick or vulnerable. I had never thought about dying or been so scared that I couldn't breathe.

I had no idea how to process the 'loss' (page 325) cancer had created across my life. I was consumed with 'anger' (page 326) and fear and had no idea how to process these feelings. I also didn't know how to create new 'meaning' (page 322) for my life post-cancer and where to place cancer within it. This was beginning to take its toll and I was losing hope.

I took a big breath and entered the support centre. And breathed. I had survived going over the threshold. I was about to do something I had never done before; ask for help. It turned out the people who ran the support centre were very willing and able to help me. It was their job to help people like me, people whose lives had been blown up by cancer and didn't know how to sort it out.

I was offered counselling. Give me anything, I didn't care, I just didn't want to feel like this. A few days later I was called by a counsellor and an appointment was made. Counselling allowed me time and space to speak freely and genuinely without fear. It was a different type of relationship and I took a different role within it. I was the vulnerable one who needed help, love and support. I wasn't being the strong, funny, crazy one now.

It was good to share my burden, really good. I was able to identify that some of my anger was about how my relationships had changed since I received the cancer diagnosis and how I was struggling with these changes. Who would I be now, carrying the heavy weight of cancer with me? After four sessions I realised these feelings were just the tip of a very large iceberg, which I was nowhere near ready to explore. I ended the sessions. I knew there was so much to come out and this terrified me. My world was already troubled. I was already struggling. I didn't need anything else to work out or manage. I couldn't cope with any more change or uncertainty. My world wasn't safe enough to explore the iceberg. So my anger remained lurking and festering. I tried to speak to the people in my life about how I felt, but they didn't understand and I suppose neither did I. I stayed connected with the centre and attended a couple of group sessions. This seemed like the right place but the wrong time for me.

THE TWO FACES OF CANCER

I associated asking for help as being a 'victim' (page 328) and failing at my 'be perfect' (page 329), 'be strong' (page 329) and 'try harder' drivers (page 329). I was overwhelmed with the 'trauma' (page 332) cancer had created and had no resilience left to work through my deep and intense feelings, so I didn't continue with the counselling.

CHAPTER 6

*"You must find the place inside yourself
where nothing is impossible."*

Deepak K. Chopra

M y hair, brows and lashes began to grow back and my body began to slowly recover from the ravages of chemo and surgery. Having had cancer, I became oversensitive and the awareness of my body and health was heightened. A cough was never just a cough, it became lung cancer; back pain was now bone cancer; lumps and bumps on my skin were now skin cancer. Anything new or different triggered the unprocessed anxiety and fear.

During these times I went back to 'stage 1' (page 317) as my 'physical dimension' (page 323) felt unsafe because of the unknown and the 'trauma' (page 332) cancer had caused. I began searching for medical reassurance that my body was safe. This turned into an 'insecure attachment' (page 317) with myself because I was constantly seeking reassurance about my health.

The anxiety migrated its way around my body visiting organs, bones and muscles in turn. I was hypervigilant and constantly scanning for the smallest of changes. I kept prodding and poking my ribs, as I was convinced I could feel something was wrong and there was something there that shouldn't be. I mentioned my discoveries to the registrar at my next check-up. I don't know what I expected him to do or not do but, quite rightly, he investigated my findings and dispatched me for an immediate X-ray. My anxiety rocketed. The X-ray had identified 'an area for concern' and I was referred for a bone scan (a scan that identifies bone abnormalities, including secondary bone cancer, which I was at risk of). I was back to being paralysed by fear again.

Because I hadn't processed my feelings about 'death' (page 321) and the previous 'trauma' (page 332), I was unable to act rationally and was immediately overwhelmed with anxiety at any trigger about ill health.

The bone scan appointment arrived, childcare was arranged and I headed back to hospital number two. Was I pregnant? I wished I was. I was given an injection of a radioactive substance from a lead syringe. I then had four hours to myself in which I was to drink as much water as possible while the radioactive stuff would head via my bloodstream and stick to any areas of bone activity indicating bone repair, damage or cancer. I had to lie still on a bed while a machine was positioned and then moved along my body collecting information. A very anxious two-week wait for the results followed.

I could not breathe for fear as I sat waiting for the appointment to receive the results, the life-changing moment when I would find out if the bone scan was clear and I could breathe again, or if I was going to be diagnosed with metastatic cancer and be a diagnosis nearer death. The scan was clear. It was suggested that I stopped prodding and poking my ribs.

The health anxiety continued. I was at the doctor's a lot, seeking reassurance for any symptom. The words offered a short and temporary relief to the anxiety. But all too soon the anxiety would return, nagging and gnawing away at me. It was an uncontainable and unmanageable situation and I felt I was constantly treading water. As with many of life's issues, external soothing rarely works and we have to learn to soothe ourselves from within. Something had to change. Over time I was able to gain some perspective and be rational, and unless a symptom was increasing or remained for more than two weeks, there was probably no reason to panic. I recognised that I was going to have to rewire my brain from a constant heightened state of alert, because feeling permanently anxious was unpleasant, pointless, all-consuming and exhausting. Every moment spent being anxious was a moment that I wasn't living and enjoying life.

Over the years (and it has taken years), I have become better at managing health anxiety. I now try to be proactive and responsible. My goal is to be aware but not worry, so I check myself over for lumps and bumps on a Monday morning in the shower. I start at my throat, working my way down and along my collar bones, breasts and armpits, as well as giving myself a quick look over for changes to moles. Doing this on a Monday means that I can take an action (that is, contact a healthcare professional) if I do discover something. If I do this on a Friday, I have to sit with the anxiety over the weekend. Rather than removing the anxiety, which is an impossible task, it's about managing the anxiety. The reality is that we all get ill at times.

> *The anxiety and feeling 'out of control' (page 333) were affecting me. I looked at what I could control and 'influence' (page 333) and channelled my energy and focus into that, so I felt I was doing what I could do, while accepting there were things I couldn't change or 'control' (page 333).*

The radiotherapy referral appointment arrived. I was on the home straight of treatment. (Radiotherapy uses radiation to destroy the cancer cells in the treated area by damaging the DNA within these cells. Although normal cells are also affected by radiation, they are better at repairing themselves than the cancer cells. Radiotherapy can be given internally or externally depending on the location of the cancer and the treatment plan).

Mrs Radiotherapy Consultant was lovely. She was a petite and elegantly-dressed lady whose clothes were so finely stitched it looked like they had been sewn by a team of fairies and hummingbirds in a Disney movie. She was gentle and kind, and felt like a soft warm blanket after the brutality of chemo and surgery. I felt safe and at ease with her, which was refreshing. In those short few moments as I held five-month-old Bonnie over my shoulder, I was brave enough to skirt around the issue of my prognosis, and before I knew it the words tumbled out. The answer she gave me has always stayed with me. She told me the tale of two of her previous patients. One had ovarian cancer who had gone on to do very well despite having a poor prognosis; and the other who had a better prognosis had been killed in a car crash on the way home from hospital. From that I drew that cancer, like life, is unpredictable and there were no guarantees. The message was loud and clear and I have not asked again.

I was still searching for someone to say the words to make my world feel safe again, to soothe my anxiety about 'death' (page 321) and uncertainty. But, of course, no one can give you a guarantee that you are going to be okay and will escape death and it was something I would have to accept in order to find peace.

I consented to treatment and was referred for the radiotherapy planning session back at hospital number three. I was starting to feel like a relay baton, being passed from person to person, hospital to hospital.

Following the surgery, and before the radiotherapy began, I had a baseline mammogram (an X-ray of the breast that is used to detect changes or breast disease), which would form a measurement against which future mammograms would be compared to identify any changes. I cannot tell you how uncomfortable the mammogram was. I have since heard it be described akin to having your boob shut in a garage door, and this is indeed an accurate description. Over the years I have developed breathing techniques to manage this.

The mammogram (and other tests) created anxiety about the unknown in my body and then about the results and the possibility of further potential 'trauma' (page 332) from a diagnosis, treatment or death.

The radiotherapy planning session involved the usual checks. I again took the familiar but reluctant half-naked position on the bed, feeling exposed and vulnerable yet again. The calculations of where the radiation would be targeted were made around and over me. There seemed to be a lot of maths involved. Co-ordinates were calculated. X-rays were taken which were used to ensure that my vital organs, such as my lungs and heart, were not in the treatment zone. I was given three further smaller tattoos called markers, which resembled blackheads in a line across my breast. These would assist the radiologists in laying me in exactly the same position to administer the treatment, ensuring the most amount of damage was caused to any remaining cancer cells and the least amount of damage to healthy cells or my lungs and heart, which were quite nearby.

The planning session was now completed, which meant one thing: I could proceed to the next challenge, twenty-five sessions of radiotherapy. The sessions ran Monday to Friday except Bank Holidays. I was given a schedule of appointment times. The next five weeks looked pretty mapped out and full-on. The staff had kindly arranged the sessions early in the day so that Ian could go to work when I got back and the girls could stay at home. Each treatment entailed a forty-mile round trip. I would leave the house at 7.30am and be back by 9.30am-ish. Sometimes, if I got back early, I would sit in the car round the corner from home, just staring out of the window because it was all I could manage. I stole time just to stare.

The radiotherapy routine was boring, monotonous and felt eternal. Get up at 6.30am, shower, eat, drive, park, walk, check in, wait, strip off, confirm who I was, lie on the couch, be positioned, be moved, be moved again and again, microscopic manoeuvers and movements until the lasers and dots confirmed I was in the right position, I was the right person in the right position, exactly the right position, exactly the position I was in yesterday, exactly the position I was going to be in tomorrow. Staff leave room, sound starts, sound ends, staff return, staff reposition me and the machine, staff leave room, sound starts, sound ends, staff come back in, get off couch, apply cream, get dressed, walk, drive, tick off another treatment, become a mum, run house, sleep. Repeat. Repeat for twenty-five days but not weekends or bank holidays. Bored. Tired. Angry.

The radiotherapy treatment room was cold and vast. In the centre was a big machine with a bed underneath it. I cried throughout the whole of the first session; silent tears of sadness fell; lonely and isolated, emotionally exhausted. And yet I kept going. I kept smiling and joking to the outside world, pretending life was okay and fun. It fucking wasn't. It was shit. I felt so exposed and vulnerable lying there.

I used a big, thick, black marker pen to cross the treatments off, as if to delete them and what the days meant to me. The days cancer robbed from me. Spring and early summer of 2004, my favourite time of year, were ruined and stolen; commuting, undressing, dressing and commuting. Fuck you cancer. The anger kept on bubbling just beneath the surface of my fake smile.

> *Letting go of further choice and time was another 'loss' (page 325) which created further 'anger' (page 326). There was no 'bargaining' (page 326) or 'denial' (page 326) at this stage; I just went to full-on anger at what I had no 'freedom' (page 322) in and what was being taken from me. It might have been helpful to 'bargain' (page 326) that I was increasing my chances of living longer.*

As the sessions progressed, the skin of the area being treated became red and itchy, and soon a perfectly formed large rectangle of red and itch began to appear. A large rectangle of red and itch marked the spot of treatment for cancer, following in the footsteps of tattoos, hair loss and scars. A dose of radiotherapy on your birthday? Or how about on your daughter's second birthday? It was rubbish. But cancer treatment marches on relentless and uncaring of special days.

The waiting rooms were packed with people older and greyer than me. The same conversations around diagnosis, treatment and session numbers whiled away the waiting.

People just like me, fearful of their future. I just wanted to be doing something else, somewhere else.

I had to take Bonnie with me to a mid-afternoon session. She was not able to remain in the room with me and I could hear her heartbreaking anguished screams of abandonment as I lay there being radiated. I felt a shit mother for having to put her through this.

The radiotherapy created intense 'isolation' (page 322). I felt disconnected from much, if not all, of my life. I was in my tenth month of treatment and had missed so much of what had continued without me. I didn't want a 'configuration of self' (page 332) as a cancer patient and I was 'angry' (page 326) at being defined as one, as well as the 'configurations of self' (page 332) which cancer had taken, and the feeling I was being seen as a 'victim' (page 328).

CHAPTER 7

"A river cuts through rock, not because of its power,
but because of its persistence."

James N. Watkins

According to the radiotherapy timetable, the treatment would end on 8th June 2004 at 8.35am. I could not wait for that day. Ten months of hell would be over and I could just return to my life and pick up where I left off. Goodbye hospital appointments. Goodbye cancer. Goodbye unpleasant thoughts and feelings. Goodbye horrible conversations. Hello life. Hello children. Hello friends. Hello carefree days. Hello choice.

Just as I had cried through the first radiotherapy session, I cried through the last, because it was over. As I dressed I felt free from the medical timetable that my life, my pregnancy and Bonnie's birth had been conducted in and around. I felt free from all that had constrained and destroyed me over the previous ten months. Just as I was thrust instantaneously into the world of cancer, I was thrust out of the medical system like a baby bird leaving the nest and having to make its own way in the world. The world which had treated me and saved me had already moved on to the next patient, called the next name.

I left the treatment room, the waiting area, the reception, the hospital, the car park. The challenges were over and the treatment complete. It was a weird feeling. A day I had craved for, and focused on for so long. There was no bouquet of flowers, no congratulatory handshake, no medal and no cheering, clapping crowd. There was no pep talk or instruction book, just another pastel-coloured leaflet to add to my collection, outlining symptoms to be aware of and the anticipated trajectory of the radiotherapy recovery.

Only it wasn't over and it never would be, but I didn't know that then. My life and world had changed, only I hadn't realised it then. I had been too occupied with surviving and ticking off treatments and appointments to think past this day.

My next challenge was to work out how my life could work again. The medical profession had done its thing. But I was left marooned and abandoned in another new and unfamiliar world. So much had changed and been lost. I knew I couldn't go back and I didn't know how to go forward. I was stuck. Although I loathed the constraints and anxiety of the hospital appointments, there was something reassuring in them, that something was being done and someone was monitoring me, treating and tracking my condition.

I now had the task of processing the 'trauma' (page 332) and 'loss' (page 325) from the last ten months and creating a new 'meaning' (page 322) to my life; something that the pastel-coloured leaflets hadn't covered. Previous life meaning had been built slowly, with changes being made over time. Change caused by cancer was big and brutal and not quickly recovered from.

In true Bex style, and not being one to miss an opportunity to party, we celebrated the end of treatment; friends, family, garden, food, fizz, smiling faces, speeches and a boob-shaped cake, reflecting on the highs and lows of the last few months. We then had a few days away with friends and I had hoped to pick my life up where I had left off. But I found it hard to enjoy anything. I was so fatigued. I could hardly look after myself, let alone function and interact with others.

The fear, anger and fatigue lingered, ruling my life now just as the hospital appointment schedule had. I faced a stark reality of life – that I was in fact not immortal and that life was not certain or guaranteed or long. You don't necessarily get to die in your seventies, eighties or nineties after you have had your life, seen your children grow up and babysat your grandchildren. I assumed that I was going to live forever, but now I wasn't sure if I was going to make it to the next Christmas. I had never actually thought about dying and what it meant. Death, like cancer, was something that happened to other people.

The 'existential given' (page 321) of 'death' (page 321) was now creating fear and feelings of being 'out of control' (page 333). My 'anger' (page 326) was now focusing on the 'loss' (page 325) of the certainty of life.

Planning anything seemed risky and potentially disappointing. I might have to cancel or postpone as cancer might call again, unannounced. I bumbled along in angry, resentful chaos. I didn't understand who I was now, what my world was. How I would crave normal, boring; a day, hour or moment free from fear.

The 'meaning' (page 322) of my life had been taken away by cancer and created 'isolation' (page 322) and disconnection from my 'social' (page 323) and 'personal' (page 324) dimensions. I knew I could not go back to this life, but because I hadn't yet worked through the impact cancer had had on me, I was unable to create new 'meaning' (page 322) to my life post-cancer. I didn't want to attach to or plan for anything in case it didn't happen or was taken away from me, and this perpetuated the cycle of 'isolation' (page 322) and disconnection.

I wanted to move on, but I didn't know how to; if I concentrated my efforts into not getting cancer again, that would be time well spent. However, cancer doesn't work in line with our previous understanding of the world; no one can prevent themselves from getting cancer. All we can do is reduce some of the risk and that leaves us with a fear we cannot fully remove, and therefore move on from, because our world can never be fully safe again.

The medical model of health and care is based on facts, figures, research and outcomes, and my treatment for cancer did not stray much from that. Self-help in the medical world focused on eating healthily, being a healthy weight, taking regular exercise, and not drinking or smoking. I wanted to do more for myself rather than feeling I was being passive and waiting for cancer to get me. I began Googling.

I was desperately searching for something I could feel I was doing and be 'in control' (page 333) of and that would help manage my anxiety when so much was 'out of control' (page 333).

My search revealed endless self-help and diet books, blogs and websites, advising many different actions and proclamations that we can prevent or even cure cancer. These ranged from cutting out food groups, silent yoga retreats or eating unusual plants grown in remote locations. Some are less scrupulous than others and I felt they were preying on scared and vulnerable people who are desperate not to be diagnosed, re-diagnosed or die from cancer. No amount of yoga, positive attitude or food choices are going to get you out of cancer. Much was moneymaking and based on personal or anecdotal evidence.

I came across The Bristol Cancer Help Centre (now Penny Brohn UK). I liked their ethos of clean living both mentally and physically. I booked a short course in late June 2004. I was still tired and without focus, willing my body to recover so I could return to life in the fast lane. The residential course was run from a delightful old house.

There were huge ceilings and large hallways containing magnificent sweeping staircases. The rooms were simply furnished with ever-changing views as the summer breeze blew the leaf-laden branches outside, revealing and then hiding the skyline. It was a gentle and supportive group environment where relaxation and a vegan diet were encouraged, neither of which I had ever tried. We did exercises to express our feelings creatively through clay and crayons. It felt good to see my feelings unfold through my hands. It felt safe. I felt understood. I was on the edge of something but not yet able to fully let myself go. There was so much to express and process. It was comforting to be among other people who knew how I was feeling. I didn't have to act or pretend. Flashes of calm and hope appeared, healing the traumas. It was a safe space to pause and reflect.

During the course I felt safe enough to reflect on what I had been through, but I didn't yet have the awareness or understanding to be able to engage with my feelings or express my 'anger' (page 326), fear and sadness at what had happened to me.

I left a few days later feeling refreshed, relaxed, calmer, less isolated and, most importantly, with a plan. I felt I was doing something outside of the medical world that I felt my life had become entrenched in. I continued with the daily meditation and would lie outside wrapped in a blanket on summer's evenings playing guided meditation CDs. The words soothed my whirring mind and my focus would be diverted away from my fear and anger. I was led up mountains, through woodlands, across fields of flowers and around blue lakes. I was frequently so exhausted that I would sleep. But I was finding an inner calm which I had been searching for, even if it wasn't for long.

I had had a really painful shoulder following the radiotherapy and, within ten days of the daily meditating, it had gone. Something was changing. I adopted a vegan diet and became slightly obsessed and uncompromising, having organic, chemical-free everything including shampoo, toothpaste and loo cleaner. I read everything around diet and cutting out milk, meat and fried food. My fear was now being managed by strict, unbreakable rules. If I couldn't control what was going on inside my body, I would take control of what I could externally. Being vegan lasted six months and I loved it, but it was tricky and time-consuming preparing three different family meals (Ian is a traditional meat and two veg man so was not interested in joining me, and I felt the girls were too young to eat a restricted diet) and socialising became a challenge. Gradually I discovered a version that fitted with my life. I became careful but not obsessed.

Time and my struggles marched on. I now hated August with a passion and was dreading the first anniversary of my cancer diagnosis: the day my life changed. The day I hate the most, with all that it means and took from me. One year on I cried many tears in the lead up to 19th August 2004. I kept replaying pre-cancer days, times and memories, and looking at photos; this time last year when life was lovely. Innocent days. It was now all so different. I wanted to mark the day, but not celebrate it. I had the most gorgeous picture taken with Poppy and Bonnie, which I still have by my bed and it's the first thing I see every morning.

They look innocent, cute and chubby; I have thick, wild and wiry hair and sadness in my eyes. A poignant day with much meaning. A day where my mind, heart and soul feel a deep and irreparable sadness. What would life have been like if cancer hadn't invaded? Another child? A mind free from anger and sadness?

The run up to the anniversary of the cancer diagnosis is always a very difficult time and triggers feelings about the 'loss' (page 325) and 'trauma' (page 332) that I experienced at the time of diagnosis.

When the active treatment ended, I was handed another pastel-coloured leaflet with symptoms to be aware of and given an appointment for a check-up in three months' time. If I remained symptom-free, the check-up period would be extended to six months in two years' time, and then annually, three years after that.

The appointments were allocated between the oncology and surgical teams. The surgical team was less able to answer my questions about current and future treatment, and would refer me to the oncology team, an appointment which could be months away. This caused me great stress and anxiety, so I asked for my care to be permanently moved to the oncology team. They were reluctant to do this, but I persevered. Learning to live with cancer was stressful enough without seeing a different medical team and them not being able to answer my questions.

Cancer had taken me emotionally back to 'stage 1' (page 317) where the world is unsafe, but unlike a young child there is no one who can make the world safe again, because ultimately no one can protect me from 'death' (page 321). My 'self-actualisation' (page 331) was driving me forward to look at what I could do to make myself feel safe and reduce the ongoing anxiety and 'trauma' (page 332) that the check-ups created by seeing different doctors each time. I felt the medical system did not meet my needs and by asking for my care to be undertaken in the oncology team, I was behaving as per 'stage 2' (page 318) and 'stage 3' (page 318) asserting my independence and needs. I did feel guilty asking for this change in care as it conflicted with my 'please others' driver (page 330).

The lead up to a test or a check-up was excruciatingly stressful and even now, fourteen years on, not much has changed. The anxiety started about a month before an appointment and increased until I was paralysed with fear. Who was I going to see? Who would look after the children? Would they let me down? What was going to be said and done? Would they find something? Would I be sent for tests? Was I going to die? The appointments and tests were triggers for the trauma I experienced during the cancer diagnosis and treatment.

The unresolved anxiety and anger continued to create a lot of internal energy which needed to be channelled. I wanted to get rid of it but, because I wasn't yet ready to engage with therapy, I kept physically busy to distract myself from these feelings. In September 2004, just three months after finishing treatment, I decided that it would be a great idea and possibly my greatest idea ever to run a marathon and raise thousands of pounds for cancer charities in the process. That would be the answer. I had never run anywhere in my life before, but I was going to do this. I would succeed and it would resolve all my issues in the process. People would marvel at the strong lady who 'beat' cancer and then ran a marathon, the perfect ending.

I had no idea how to end with cancer or where to place it within my life. If I invented a happy ending where I succeeded in achieving something, I would feel less of a failure for having cancer in the first place and not being a good mum while I had the treatment.

I bought trainers, joined a running club and began running. This would be fun. I was still recovering from treatment but pushed on relentlessly, not listening to my body. My lungs heaved as I dragged my unfit and unwilling body along pavements, mile after mile. Others who were considerably fitter than me and who hadn't just had ten months of cancer treatment, and who had run for years, chatted away around me. It all looked so easy, why was it so hard for me? My mind wanted to do something, but my body had very different ideas. It screamed for me to stop and eventually I did. I gave up running and my marathon plans. Running a marathon was not the answer.

I was searching for a way to create 'meaning' (page 322) in my life again and feel 'in control' (page 333). Running was a way of channelling the feelings, which I found very uncomfortable to experience but had no strategy to deal with. My 'self-actualisation' (page 331) was trying new things to see if they would resolve the situation as per 'stage 4' (page 318) and 'stage 5' (page 319).

Bonnie's first birthday in October marked a celebration of life; a life with a precarious beginning, a life which had been jeopardised because of my choices. We celebrated with her friends, we celebrated with her family, and we celebrated with her. We appreciated what we have because it could have all been so very different. We appreciated that she is safe and well, and that I am safe and well. I think back to the day I first met her, and what a miracle she was; the tiny bundle of hope, and all she meant to me and all she had been through. She was part of that difficult journey with me; my guilt that she had no choice, a captive in my belly.

I bumped and bungled my way through the remainder of 2004, functioning but feeling lost, isolated and disconnected. This was interspersed with outbursts of energy and anger. It was good to leave the year behind. It became the year my cancer treatment ended, and 2005 was new and fresh and untainted.

Early in 2005 I felt suddenly unwell and developed flu. I was really ill for weeks. My body was not recovered from the cancer treatment and had nothing left to give. I started coughing and was still coughing some eight weeks later. I just couldn't shake the cough off. I knew some sunshine would do the trick and so booked a few days away with Poppy in the Canary Islands. I was terrified and hesitant as I said goodbye to Ian and Bonnie at border control. But it was so lovely to have Poppy to myself; my eyes, thoughts and feelings just focusing on her once more. The trip was just what I needed: warmth, sunshine, a beautiful beach and an all-inclusive buffet. The cough cleared. It was lovely to spend some quality, relaxing time with just Poppy. Gradually the broken bonds began to repair. I watched Poppy paddle in the shallow blue pool and take large bowlfuls of olives from the buffet, her cheeky grin gaining my attention once more. I watched her sleep, looking minute in the large king-sized bed next to me. We pottered and played, walked along the sandy beach and drank mocktails on trendy white sofas, watching the sunset; chattering away; smiling; being each other's focus once more; me loving her; her loving me.

This trip repaired some of the guilt I experienced at not being there or being available physically or emotionally to Poppy while I was having the cancer treatment.

CHAPTER 8

"You are never too old to set another goal
or to dream a new dream."

C.S. Lewis

Bit by bit my physical health and spirit began to return. Although life was clearly never going to be the same, I had a life and it was up to me to live it. I continued to grieve the loss of certainty of life and having more children. The thoughts of not being there to see my children grow up, and not to be able to protect them from death, whirred away in my head. I continued to spend time spinning from being manic and angry to avoid engaging with and working through the thoughts and feelings cancer had created.

Over time my trust in life returned and I felt safe again, but I was still grieving for the 'loss' (page 325) of many things. As I became less stressed, I began to realise it was my responsibility to lead a life which was 'meaningful' (page 322) to me and I had 'freedom' (page 322) to choose this. I hadn't got to 'acceptance' (page 327) about the finiteness of time and life, and leaving my children and being a good mum felt like 'unfinished business' (page 331), especially while the girls were so young. I was experiencing conflict between my 'configuration of self' (page 332) of being a good mum and being there unfailingly for my children, and 'death' (page 321) – I had yet to find a place where I could balance the two.

Cancer robbed me of my already fragile confidence. I was now walking around looking dowdy and androgynous, my head and face permanently facing down. If I hid, cancer may not find me again. A friend knew I had always wanted a colour analysis to find out which colours suit me best and booked me an appointment with an image consultant. The image consultant draped various coloured scarves over my jaw line (okay it was a tad more technical than this) declaring I was a 'summer' pallet. It was so fascinating to see how the correct shade of a colour can change how we look, and in turn how we feel and behave. I was hooked.

The next step was to analyse my body shape and discover what style of clothes suit me. Basically I am shaped like a brick, with good limbs, a dodgy tummy area and no waist. Plain clothes with a dash of daring suit me best. The image consultant came to my home, where we worked through my wardrobe deciding what should be kept, altered or dumped. It was cathartic and refreshing. My wardrobe looked empty after this process; an eclectic mix of coat hangers remained waiting for a new identity to be hung on them, much like where I found myself in the post-cancer wasteland. We then went shopping to buy my new look. It was fun to try on and then buy the outfits suggested by her, many of which I would never have chosen myself. She was a great boost for my confidence. Over the years, my image consultant has created a subtly changing look and has remained my personal shopper ever since. I don't spend a fortune and I shop in high street chains, but what has changed is that I now know I look the best I can and this has created an air of inner confidence.

The shopping trips repaired and built my sense of confidence and created a new part of my post-cancer 'configuration of self' (page 332) and identity as per 'stage 5' (page 319). I knew I looked good and in turn felt good.

The months of isolation I experienced during the treatment and recovery from cancer was excruciating and drove me slightly crazy. I wanted to fire up an imaginary chainsaw and begin slaying what was wrong with my life, except I didn't know what it was that needed slaying or where to begin. I was still swinging from angry to depressed or anxious, and right back round again. I hadn't experienced anything like this in my life. As no one I knew had experienced anything remotely similar, I didn't feel that anyone would understand my fear, my sadness or my anger. I felt I had little in common with my friends. They were enjoying their lives, new babies, toddler mornings, trips to the swings, feeding the ducks – while I felt detached, disconnected and out of control.

Because I was young and pregnant when I was diagnosed, I didn't feel I identified with many people who I met along the way either. The people I met were generally much older and worried about not seeing their grandchildren grow up. I just wanted to see my children into their primary school. Their worries and focus were different. I felt I stood out; my attachments and sense of belonging shattered. From this place of isolation, something began to burn in me that I wanted to help lessen the isolation for other people who faced similar experiences, by using my own experiences; an altruistic thought which began to grow.

> *I hadn't found anyone who could 'rescue' (page 328) me from my feelings of 'isolation' (page 322) and 'trauma' (page 332), so I began looking to 'rescue' (page 328) others instead. I was still avoiding my feelings and used this as a way to continue to do so; if I was helping others I wouldn't have to face my own feelings. However, this was the beginning of finding 'meaning' (page 322) to my life, my 'configuration of self' (page 332), 'social' (page 323) and 'personal' (page 324) dimensions post-cancer.*

Despite having lots of good and happy things, people and events in my life, my needs around recovering emotionally and psychologically from cancer were not being met, mainly because I was avoiding the enormity of them. The support groups and counselling had not addressed what I needed. During one random Google-searching session, I stumbled upon a UK-based charity called Breast Cancer Care.

Breast Cancer Care offers a wide range of services to anyone affected by breast cancer. I clicked around the website until I found an online forum. I *loved* that online forum. I stayed on there for hours feeding and distracting the girls while reading the threads and posts over and over again. Finally I had hit what felt like the jackpot of support. This was perfect for me. I could be anonymous. I could access it from home twenty-four hours a day while the girls slept or played. I didn't have to arrange childcare or put on a brave face or drive twenty miles. It was there continuously, updating constantly on the screen in front of my eyes.

I could gain and give support, read rants and write rants, understand and be understood, and at long last I finally felt less isolated. I was not the only young mum diagnosed with cancer, scared and angry, alone and isolated, juggling children and appointments, listening to crass comments and intrusive questions. Log-in names hid treatment plans, locations and identities. I spent many hours on the online forum feeling connected and safe. We all spoke the same language and shared the same feelings. I loved reading people moaning about doctors and insensitive comments from others. I also loved offering words of encouragement to those just starting on this hellish journey. I identified with the fears and concerns because I knew, I really knew, how they felt. The forum saved my life emotionally, just as my oncologist had saved it physically.

The online forum created a connection, which instantly lessoned the intense 'isolation' (page 322) I had been experiencing. Because I felt safe on the forum I was able to express myself freely and feel

understood, and I was able to build on 'stage 1' (page
317). The world began to feel safe again, which meant
I could move on.

I began to feel very connected to the charity and the work
they undertook. I began to work as a media volunteer for
Breast Cancer Care and did many TV, radio and magazine
interviews and photo shoots, both with and without the
girls. We would travel to London and arrive at airy loft
house studios on leafy streets. The rooms would be filled
by trendy young stylists who would fuss over us. We would
be groomed, styled and photographed, looking the picture
of health and happiness, telling our story of triumph
over disaster and raising awareness of breast cancer. I
hoped I would help someone else facing those difficult
conversations and treatments to believe they could get
through cancer, just as I had. I of course glossed over the
fact that cancer drove me to the brink of my mental health
and I still wasn't anywhere near recovered, emotionally or
psychologically. These media events helped me to use my
cancer experience in a positive way. That sounds so crass,
but I was finding how and where to place cancer and its
impact on my life. I was still connected to cancer, but it
wasn't wounding or debilitating me. It was beginning to
have a place and a purpose.

I was now finding a place for my cancer experience
and trying out new roles, as in 'stage 5' (page 319).
I knew I could not delete cancer from my life and
wanted to use it in a positive way that had 'meaning'
(page 322) and healing for me. This was driven by

both my 'rescuer' (page 328), to lessen the 'isolation' (page 322) for others, and my 'self-actualisation' (page 331) which drove me forward to feel happy again and close the 'unfinished business' (page 331) cancer had left me with. The volunteer work built my confidence because I felt both empowered and 'in control' (page 333) of my choices. By telling my cancer story I was able to process the feelings and 'trauma' (page 332) it had created.

Being active in raising awareness of breast cancer felt good and I am still an avid campaigner. But there was still a passion, a drive that was not being met. I knew this was the right area of work, but the wrong role within it. Once I had reached two years after my diagnosis, I was eligible to apply to be a peer supporter at Breast Cancer Care. If I was successful in my application and training, I would provide telephone support to other women who faced a similar experience. I applied for the role with excitement and was delighted to be successful. I felt I was moving in the right direction and felt very supported by Breast Cancer Care in the training and in the role. I was matched with several ladies over a couple of years, supporting them through their diagnosis, treatment and recovery. Again, it was a positive step and experience, but still not quite right. The role gave me confidence that I was on the right track and the next step was to find some formal training.

The role with the charity helped me build my confidence and a 'configuration of self' (page 332) as a helper was emerging. I was at 'stage 4' (page

318), gaining confidence, and 'stage 5' (page 319), exploring who I was post-cancer treatment. There was still an unmet need and my 'self-actualisation' (page 331) kept driving me forward until I found it.

During this time, I returned to the cancer support centre where I'd had my first taste of counselling. I became involved as a volunteer and trustee. Again, this satisfied my needs for a while, but the familiar pattern returned and in time the role didn't feel right. I still wanted something else, but was getting closer each time.

The need this time was channelled into setting up a charity to support women who are diagnosed with cancer during pregnancy. Support for Cancer in Pregnancy was conceived. I had a logo designed and built a website. Using my feelings in this way was much less destructive; they had a place to go and a purpose. I was finding my way and it was freeing to my mind. I felt connected and passionate about the work I was doing and the support I was giving. The desire to lessen the isolation for others grew in line with my returning confidence and energy. The anger and anxiety were now passion and drive, and were channelled into my charity work. Over the coming weeks and months I did some valuable work and supported a few ladies through their diagnosis, treatment and recovery, using the skills learned and experiences from my cancer, Breast Cancer Care and the cancer support centre. I found supporting other people incredibly rewarding, but I wanted to do it better and began to consider formally training as a counsellor.

As I found ways to channel my cancer experience, the 'anger' (page 326) lessened. I was still trying out the roles in 'stage 5' (page 319) to find the right role and this need remained 'unfinished business' (page 331) until I had.

In October 2007 I began an Introduction to Counselling course. It was basic but enjoyable, and necessary if training as a counsellor was where I wanted to go. The wasteland which my life had become post-cancer now had the beginnings of very small and very fragile, but very bright green shoots.

My life was beginning to take focus and shape, incorporating my experience of cancer to create 'meaning' (page 322) in my 'personal' (page 324) and 'spiritual' (page 324) dimensions and to address the 'loss' (page 325) and 'isolation' (page 322) in my 'social dimension' (page 323) that cancer had caused.

It was also at this time that I resumed having counselling sessions myself again. These sessions ended up lasting ten years. Initially the sessions focused on my relationship with Ian, because that was not running smoothly – maybe not surprisingly after two children and a diagnosis of cancer arriving within sixteen months, as well as the highs and lows of family life and running your own business. There had been too much trauma and change. Ian is a business risk-taker and works on cycles of boom and bust, feast and famine. I kept things stable at home to counteract this, but this was not possible with what I had been through and things were rocky.

My counsellor created a safe and trusting space for me to crash around in; to cry, explore, be frustrated, and be supported. She was understanding and caring. She supported me through the dramas, tears, avoidance, frustration, awareness and change. She challenged me just the right amount, in just the right way, at just the right time. She knows my whole story: the dark and dingy corners; the choices; the behaviours that I am not proud of, that I am mortified about and ashamed of; Where I felt fucked up; where I felt fucked over; where I fucked others over; where I should have been kinder or stronger. She accepted all of those while I worked it out for myself, while I worked out who I was. Cancer gave me the reason and motivation to change and my counsellor gave the support with which to do so. She did not give up on me. She waited with me; a safe, secure and stable attachment in the chaos of my life.

Through therapy I gained awareness and, in time, choice as I looked at my life and myself one small chunk at a time. I became aware of my repetitive dysfunctional behaviours and thought processes, the triggers and outcomes. At times it was unbearable and terrifying, but I stayed with the process. I kept going, driven by the thought of finding out who I was and how I could lead a happy and satisfying life. But that meant change and letting go of relationships, thoughts, feelings and behaviours. I began to make small changes. I stopped running and fighting. I became less angry, less caught up in the creation of and involvement in dramas, and in time was able to accept help, love and eventually myself. I let go of the views that others had imposed on me and I let go of the expectations others had of me; the views and expectations that created resentment and frustration in me, trying to live in them and up to them to keep other people happy, at the cost of my own happiness. It was tough and required honesty, openness, resilience, commitment, hard work and the crying of many, many tears. I let go of so much and at one point did not know who I was anymore.

Gradually, I began to like and value myself. My counsellor re-parented me so I could parent myself. The dramas that I created wherever I went were a defence against exploring pain from the past, a temporary relief from the years of emotional pain that I carried around with me. I bored myself in the end with my behaviour; the same words, the same actions, the same outcomes, the same consequences. I was exhausted with being a rebel, pushing the boundaries and seeking attention. I wanted to live my life quietly and calmly in a deeper, more satisfying and meaningful way. I didn't want to leave my life as a string of texts or social media posts about the latest calamity or crazy idea. I needed to change. I wanted to change. And, through counselling, I changed.

A new tentatively assertive Rebecca was emerging. Some people loved her and plenty didn't, but I was beginning to care less and less. I now knew what my values in life were and I was increasingly confident in recognising and expressing these. I felt I was hurting and rejecting people who had been in my life for years, but I kept going because I believed what I was doing was right for me.

The work was as fascinating as it was difficult. When I finished my sessions it was like a bereavement. It was the right choice to finish when I did but it hurt for a while.

Counselling provided a stable and safe space for me to explore myself and create a 'secure attachment' (page 316) with myself and, in time, others. I knew I was not living the life I wanted to and my 'self-actualisation' (page 331) and 'try harder' (page 329) driver drove me to find change and kept me going when the going got tough. My 'configurations of self' (page 332) changed a lot during this time, with some receding and others emerging, and this was uncomfortable. My 'be perfect' (page 329) driver fought the change because she wanted to avoid being vulnerable.

CHAPTER 9

"You can't put a limit on anything.
The more you dream, the farther you get."

Michael Phelps

O nce the active cancer treatment had finished, I was keen never to return voluntarily to a hospital again. I had had enough of being prodded, poked, examined, discussed and tested. I wanted my life back. My small, scarred breast was an insignificant price to pay to have my life back. I rarely looked in the mirror naked in order to avoid having to engage with the image I would see. About six years after my diagnosis, in 2009, as I took a peak at my scarred and uneven body, I began to wonder about reconstructive surgery. I had always been an 'A' cup and had never felt I had a feminine body. I wondered about reconstructive surgery and tentatively asked about it at my next check-up. I was referred on to a specialist plastic surgery hospital.

I casually went to the appointment at hospital number four with an expectation that nothing could be done and it was more about ruling reconstruction out than in. I was surprised therefore when the consultant said I would be suitable for reconstructive surgery, suggesting a 'D' cup breast size would suit me. He went on to say that the surgery could take place six weeks later.

I quickly gathered together my thoughts as they whizzed around my excited brain at an increasing pace. The plan was to insert two different sized silicone implants to even up and enlarge my breast size. In no time at all I was happily signing a consent form. This consent form was different – it felt exciting, empowering and positive. Ian and I laughed as we put rice-filled plastic bags into a bra to calculate the right volume for the implants. Very precise and technical, I thought. I was blasé about the side effects and risks as I was enjoying the feelings of choice and control.

In my process of 'bargaining' (page 326) about cancer, and that I was alive and could be with my girls, I avoided thinking about how the brutality of breast cancer surgery and my differing breast sizes had damaged my self-confidence and my feminine 'configuration of self' (page 332). Breast reconstruction felt like a positive step in building and rebuilding my self-confidence and sense of self following cancer, and was something I felt 'in control' (page 333) of.

This surgery kit list involved a sports bra in the new cup size and front-opening tops. I gave both negligible thought. It was nice to buy and pack the kit list this time, with feelings of excitement and optimism rather than fear and sadness. We set off for the hospital and checked in. I giggled as the big black pen tickled my body as it was marked up for surgery. And then, a blank of time as the surgical team did their thing. As I came round slowly from the anaesthetic in the recovery room I reached up and touched my breasts, slurring to the nurse that I was just checking I had what I had come in for. They were enormous. I loved them already. Although the drains were back, this felt so different, positive, whereas after the other surgeries I had felt panicky at what the outcome would be. I was returned to the ward, groggy and sleepy. My face lit up when Ian and the girls came back to visit later in the day. Bonnie had lost a tooth, having being hit in the mouth by a swing; her face was red and swollen from the impact. I smiled and was glad life was continuing normally for them.

My new breasts were not only very large, but also very sore and tender. Even just a sheet laid over them was uncomfortable. Following the surgeon's check the next day, I was eased into the sports bra, which I would wear for twenty-four hours a day for the next six weeks. The bra had looked enormous when I bought it, but it was now very tight and I felt trussed up like a chicken ready for roasting.

I had casually listened to the run through of the side effects and risks prior to surgery, but no one could convey the odd feelings which followed the surgery. During the next few days I was extremely uncomfortable, sore and stiff everywhere. Holding a drink was a challenge and hair washing was out. I could not lift my arms as they had no strength, and it was then I knew why front-opening tops had been recommended. I was constantly waiting for pain relief to arrive, tracking the trolley as it inched nearer. Gradually a bruise appeared, from my breast to my hip, faint at first but changing colours, tones and shades through blue, black, green and yellow, and eventually fading away.

I ate and slept and pottered round the hospital. The time soon passed and I was discharged six days later. Life was lived at a slower pace while my body repaired and recovered.

Gradually I recovered, over a period of about four weeks. The swelling reduced, the bruising faded, the movement returned. I brought new bras and tops and began to enjoy my new look and bigger boobs. The new, bigger, better boobs are not symmetrical or perfect, and the breast cancer scar is still there, but clothed I felt confident and feminine. I began to like how I looked for the first time in my life and my mental health took a step forward. I still find it hard to look at myself naked in front of the mirror. The reflection shows the scars, the reasons, the memories, but clothed I feel good.

The breast enlargement created a 'configuration of self' (page 332) of feeling feminine, which in turn built my self-confidence.

My counsellor had encouraged me to take photos before and after the reconstructive surgery. I was reluctant and resisted because I hated how I looked; the scarring and the unfeminine shape. But I trusted her in seeing the bigger picture and I'm glad I did. Those pictures are hard to look at, but they are a visual record of part of my life; the part in the middle, after I was smooth and perfect, and before I was feminine and confident.

CHAPTER 10

"I don't want to get to the end of my life
and find that I just lived the length of it.
I want to have lived the width of it as well."

Diane Ackerman

Through therapy I was able to work through my thoughts and feelings, and this freed me to begin to think about other things. Time became a focus for me: how I used time, the passage of time, the amount of time left and the end of my time (I have explored my thoughts about death in more depth in chapter 25). The problem with time is we don't know when it will run out, and cancer had given me a taster of what that feels like and it was frightening. Over time, I was able to trust there may be more time available to me and to think further ahead than the next two hours. Time became an important and precious commodity for me. I now knew health, life and time was limited and wanted to use what was left to me wisely. I began to be more focused and, in some ways, selfish with my time. If I wasn't doing all the crazy shit, I could spend time doing things that had meaning to me and gave me satisfaction, things that I would look back on and be proud of. I started to think about what I wanted to achieve and began compiling a bucket list, with the aim of achieving one item a year.

My bucket list wasn't just an idle list of maybes. Each item had been thought about. Each item had meaning. Each item was a goal I wanted to achieve. Each item was a 'fuck you' to cancer. Each item gave me hope when there wasn't any. Each item created motivation and control over what I couldn't control. My bucket list created a focus on the future and something to look forward to, to hope for. My bucket list created a relief from the psychological anxiety I was experiencing around death; if I'm living and achieving my list, I'm not worrying or thinking about dying.

My first bucket list looked like this:

1. Take Bonnie to school on her first day. (This had been my motivation to keep going when, during the winter of 2003, I felt so hopeless I didn't think I could go on.)
2. Travel to Australia. (I was not confident enough to travel the world when I was younger and felt this was an unfulfilled part of my life, and this again had kept my focus on life during the winter of 2003 when I didn't think I could go on.)
3. Have a trip in a hot air balloon. (I had always wondered what the world would look like from the sky.)

4. Go to an airshow. (I was fascinated with planes. How could something so big and heavy fly? I wanted a closer look.)
5. Go to a music festival. (I loved music and camping, and wanted to experience the sights and sounds of a festival.)
6. Visit the Polish National Horse Show. (I love Polish Arabian horses and wanted to visit the country and studs which bred them.)
7. See Madonna in concert. (I loved the rebelliousness of Madonna and found her fascinating, and wanted to see one of her live shows.)
8. Drive a tractor. (I had seen many tractors during my country living and horse days, and wondered what it would be like to drive something so big, something slightly dangerous and therefore exciting.)
9. Travel to Kerala. (I loved heat, people, colour and korma, had seen Kerala on a travel show and was captivated by its beauty.)
10. Have a career (I had not been to university or had a career, and I regretted this.)

The two bucket list items which had the most meaning were taking Bonnie to school on her first day and visiting Australia.

In the long, desolate, winter days of 2003 there were times when I didn't feel I could go on. I felt totally hopeless. I would force myself out of bed and resist the urge to return there at numerous points throughout the day. I just wanted to wait in bed until this hell was over, hiding under the duvet while cancer just happened around me; safe, unconscious and unaware; no more treatment, no more trauma, no one would know I was there if I kept quiet and still enough. My brain wouldn't have to take in, process and action anything else; no more choice; no more struggle; escaping the effort I had to put in just to survive each hour, each day, each decision, each appointment, each treatment; just getting to the end of a day; just getting to the next nappy change, bottle mix, bath and bedtime; just getting through the next two hours; the next two hours were doable, manageable.

When my thoughts and feelings would overwhelm me and I didn't think I could carry on, I would ask myself the same question: 'Do you want to take Bonnie to school on her first day?' The answer was always yes, so I would get up, attend the next appointment, have the next treatment. That question was my motivator, and at times still is. My girls, my gorgeous girls, who I could not protect from any of this cancer hell, motivated me to carry on and be their mum when I really didn't think I could.

Bonnie grew and appeared to follow a normal development trajectory. Feisty and determined, with a brain and thought process which fascinated me on a daily basis. By three she had sussed that Father Christmas did not exist. By five she wanted to perform post-mortems on dead animals 'to see how they worked' and exhume dead pets to 'see what happened'. Her observations and view of the world was intriguing and her questions relentless, and many of which I couldn't answer. She wanted to design a round crisp packet so that bits wouldn't gather in the corner. She would wear the same outfit for days on end; freeing her mind of choice so it could observe and wonder. She knows what she does and doesn't like, and what she does and doesn't want, and can communicate her needs, sometimes very clearly and loudly without compromise. I have never met anyone with such a strong sense of self.

Poppy in contrast was quiet and introverted, sweet and soft. She began pre-school at three and was mute for most of her year there, still cautious of new settings after the chaos that cancer had brought to her world. She started school looking tiny in her uniform and only found her feet from year two onwards. She is wise, determined and empathic, with nerves of steel.

Bonnie began pre-school the day Poppy started school, so starting school was still two years away for her. It was a milestone which felt precarious and fragile, would I make it? Would it get tantalisingly close, only to be taken away? I marched on through the fog of unprocessed feelings towards the possibility of this day. As the days and months progressed, there was an increasing chance I would be here to take Bonnie to school on her first day. Cautiously, and not assuming or taking anything for granted, I began to focus on this day with increasing determination and energy. No matter how it took place, I was taking Bonnie to school on her first day.

The school application; the visits; the letter offering a place; leaving pre-school; July, August, the beginning of September; the uniform, shoes, kit list, labelling the night before; the day; the dawn; the hour; the minute; the car journey; the school playground; the wave goodbye. I had made it. I was alive. I had lived to take Bonnie to school on her first day. That cute blonde-haired girl who had unwittingly and unknowingly come along with me for two cycles of the chemo was walking up the path to her first day at school, happy, healthy and blissfully unaware, just as it should be. She had kept me focused, she had kept me determined.

The joy and utter relief that I was alive and healthy to witness this day was immense. In my mind there were flags, bunting and glasses of champagne everywhere. If I had dropped down dead at this point it would have been okay. I enjoyed the moment but, as it became the past, my mind was soon racing on to the next focus, the next goal. Would I see her out of primary school or should I aim further ahead, out of secondary school or to university? First job, first boyfriend, first broken heart? Backpacking trip, tattoo, driving lesson, wedding or baby? It's these landmark dates and events that I appreciate and cherish because I don't assume or take for granted that I will be alive to see them.

During the long, hopeless days of 2003 I began to think about Australia, a country I had never visited. It sounded distant and different. My vision was that one day I would go with the girls, when Poppy was ten. Life was so impossibly hard, and yet this vision was so clear, so definite. When I was having negative moments, moments of overwhelming fear and hopelessness, moments when there was no future, I would visualise this trip.

Unexpectedly, in April 2011, Lovely Brother started a three-year work secondment in Sydney and would be packing up with his family and moving to the other side of the world. I was so sad to see them go and booked myself a week in August 2011 to visit them. August soon came around and I excitedly set off on my own mini-adventure. It was scary, but exciting and liberating. It was 'fuck you' and 'thank you' cancer. The sun was rising as the flight path took us over Sydney Harbour and I gained my first sight of Sydney. I was in love with this cosmopolitan city before I had landed. It was good to catch up with Lovely Brother and his family, comforting to see them in their house, and experience fragments of their lives.

Over the next few days, I enjoyed the beaches, coastal walks, food, cafés, outdoor lifestyle and iconic buildings. We ate dinner in stylish restaurants and sipped cocktails in swish bars. I travelled to Manly Beach by ferry across the harbour, feeling free from the negativity, struggles and restraint that cancer had brought to my life. This was a time to enjoy and savour. We saw an opera at the Opera House. We travelled to the Blue Mountains, just outside Sydney, passing kangaroos along the roadside. The vastness of this country struck me as we enjoyed the spectacular panoramic views of the eucalyptus forests beneath us covered in a blue haze. I cherished each and every moment.

I was sad to leave Sydney at the end of my week, but I was now even more passionate and determined about us all going to Australia and we travelled back there as a family in December 2012 to spend Christmas and New Year there. This was a dream come true. I savoured the planning and packing, the shopping and the preparation. The flight was long but I didn't care. I was living a dream which had kept me going when my world was bleak and hopeless. We arrived in Sydney looking pale and washed out early in December. We spent an idyllic few days in Sydney to recover. I loved watching the cousins play together like lion cubs. I sat listening to the waves crash in on Maroubra Beach, the children noisily catching fish in the rock pools nearby, watching surfers waiting patiently in the distance for the perfect wave to ride back to shore on. I pondered the enormity of a land so far away from home, a reality far away from the desperate dream I had thought about endlessly during the nightmare of cancer.

We then flew to Noosa, further up the eastern coast of Australia, for a week. We rented a waterfront apartment. Noosa has a gorgeous beach, chic shops and the constant noise of the ocean. I cried leaving there as it was just so lovely. We travelled back to Sydney via the stunning Blue Mountains, returning to Sydney for Christmas and New Year. It was different being so far away from home on Christmas Day, but we ate turkey and Brussels sprouts and it rained all day so it felt like a home from home.

The highlight of the trip was spending New Year's Eve on a beautiful boat moored in Sydney Harbour, with uninterrupted views of the Opera House and Harbour Bridge. We packed up a seafood and champagne picnic and made our way to the boat mooring in the early evening to be sure of getting a good position. The sun began to set and the noise from the boats around us grew, as did the atmosphere, as we got nearer to the New Year. Out of the darkness Kylie's voice began counting down and our eyes focused on the Harbour Bridge, which became a riot of noise and colour in the darkness of the night. I had to pinch myself that this was really happening and I was really there. It was incredible. The fireworks, the iconic location, the atmosphere and noises all created a moment in time such that if I had died on the way back, it wouldn't have mattered. A New Year to remember. I had made it. Death and cancer hadn't caught up with me just yet.

We left to return to the UK in early January. I had a

sad but satisfied heart. I had appreciated and enjoyed every single second we were there because it was a dream come true, dreamt up during a time when there was really no hope.

Bonnie's first day at school and the trip to Australia will always be my most precious and meaningful memories, because they had created focus and hope when I couldn't see or feel either.

I had faced the 'existential given' (page 321) of 'death' (page 321) and experienced intense 'isolation' (page 322) and multiple 'loss' (page 325) during my cancer diagnosis, treatment and recovery. I was now beginning to rebuild my life by revising it's 'meaning' (page 322) post-cancer through my bucket list, which in turn impacted on my 'social' (page 323), 'personal' (page 324) and 'spiritual' (page 324) dimensions. I strove to achieve my bucket list because of the reality of 'death' (page 321) which I can't avoid, but I can create 'meaning' (page 322) in my life through the choices I make between now and then.

Achieving these goals and experiences was an important part of my emotional and psychological recovery from cancer. I was finding out who I would be post-cancer as well as learning to live with the unpredictability of cancer. Achieving the bucket list built my confidence, which had been lost during cancer, as well as creating feelings of being 'in control' (page 333). My 'self-actualisation' (page 331) drove me relentlessly to achieve and create a life with 'meaning' (page 322). Realising the finiteness of time, health and life, my 'hurry up' driver (page 330) created impatience and frustration if even a minute of time was wasted.

I became aware that my 'configuration of self' (page 332) of being scared was being counteracted by the 'configuration of self' (page 332) of being a rebel, and because I was desperate not to be seen as a 'victim' (page 328), I would do attention-seeking things as a distraction so people would focus on my achievements and not see me as a cancer patient.

My bucket list remained an important focus for me. However, it came with consequences and at times it created guilt in my pursuit of it. I'm not a big one for guilt. In fact it's a feeling I rarely feel. So much so that during my counselling training I read a book about it, as I just did not identify with the feeling. I do, however, feel massively guilty about leaving the girls. I was so unavailable to them while I was being treated for cancer that this has left a lasting scar which is retriggered if I leave them to go and do something for me. I didn't have a choice about leaving them for treatment, I had to go, but I do have a choice to leave them now and that presents me with a dilemma. It is a dilemma driven by the deeply painful thought that one day we will be separated permanently by death and until then I want to spend every second I can with them. It is a dilemma of wanting to see, explore and experience the world before time and health runs out, and I want to share this passion and these experiences with the girls. I want to travel to far-flung places to experience cultures, spices, endless sandy beaches lapped by clear, pristine seas, boat trips, architecture, languages, jet lag, dodgy showers and hot sweaty train journeys. As the girls have got older they don't want the same kind of holidays as I do, and so I have had to acknowledge and respect that they don't have the same views, desires or urgency as me. For them time is not a limited commodity.

I feel grateful that we did a lot of trips and travels together while they were younger, more malleable and willing to spending endless hours at 35,000 feet so I could tick something off my bucket list. We have had quality time, adventures and experiences together, and I hope one day they will share my sense of adventure in this wonderful world.

Not providing my 'configuration of self' (page 332) as a mum is something I find very difficult and forms part of the 'loss' (page 325) I experienced in knowing that one day I will have to. By creating memories I am avoiding this and lessening the 'unfinished business' (page 331) from 'stage 8' (page 319) for myself. By doing so much with the girls, over time I have repaired the guilt and 'loss' (page 325) I experienced at not living up to my 'be perfect' driver (page 329) and 'configuration of self' (page 332) of being the perfect mum. Each choice I make has a consequence. If I don't travel I feel resentment at not going and have 'unfinished business' (page 331) of wanting to see places and have experiences. But if I go, I feel guilty at leaving the girls, and if I make them go with me I'm not respecting their choice and feel guilty for that too.

I have been the focus of some jealousy and envy from

people because of the things I have done and I fully appreciate that I have been very fortunate to be able to do some wonderful things. The pay-off (which may be unseen for some) is that I live with the daily knowledge and fear that one day I won't have my health, life or choice, because I will be too ill, and time and life will have passed me by. I am aware that each and every life has an end point, but I have an urgency to dream, to achieve, to live, to complete. I don't take for granted that I will have years of health and life ahead of me in which to achieve them.

This is probably the only good thing to come out of having cancer, to live my life in a satisfying and 'meaningful' (page 322) way and to regularly reflect on and then action 'stage 8' (page 319).

CHAPTER 11

"Do the best you can until you know better.
Then when you know better, do better."

Maya Angelou

With Poppy and now Bonnie settled into school, a large void appeared in my life. The energy and focus I had put into the goal of being there to take Bonnie to school needed to be channelled elsewhere. The next step was about engaging my brain again. I saw a part-time job advertised in the shop window at a local events company as we drove past returning from a summer holiday. I loved organising and people. I stopped the car, grabbed the details and speedily scrambled my CV together, sending it in nervously with a covering letter. I was interviewed and offered a post which fitted around the girls' school hours.

Although I had identified some of my feelings around the 'loss' (page 325) and 'trauma' (page 332) of cancer, I had nowhere near begun to work my way through them; I was still looking for things to distract myself and keeping myself constantly busy so I wouldn't have to address them.

While I was working part-time, and having passed the Introduction to Counselling Course, I began the next stage of counselling training in January, with a Certificate in Counselling. I found the course both challenging and fascinating. I loved learning about counselling theory; it created understanding about myself, and I began to recognise I had a flair for working with people. I liked them, I got on with them and I understood them. My energy and focus were being channelled in the right way. If I passed this course it would give me access to begin a foundation degree in counselling, in September. The drive to help people and create change hadn't diminished, the passion was still bubbling away; I now had time to focus, and gradually I was beginning to realise I had the skills as well. I studied hard, completing the tasks both in and out of lesson time. Practising skills and writing a reflective diary, it felt good to say the things I had been carrying around with me for so long, burdening me, weighing me down.

With relief and pride, I passed the Certificate in Counselling Course and applied for the humanistic route for the foundation degree. After submitting the application form and accompanying written work, I attended a group interview. Much was riding on this, and I was nervous. I really wanted this. I regretted not having a degree. I passed and was accepted along with twenty-three other trainee counsellors, each with their own reason for starting the course.

At the ripe old age of forty-four I began training as a counsellor and studying for a degree. I was happy, excited and proud. I had wanted both for a while and so was dedicated and focused. I had found something I was passionate about and determined to complete, and this saw me through the challenging times that lay ahead during the course. It was constantly absorbing, demanding and challenging. During the three-year course there were essays and deadlines, theories to understand and apply, personal therapy, professional development, ethical practice, clinical placements to arrange, and presentations to research. Throughout, we received cutting feedback and reflections about ourselves from our peers and tutors, and at times our clients. It was harsh. I could either be damaged by it or I could learn from it. I chose the latter.

Just as cancer changed everything, so did the counselling course. The course content was designed to challenge, question, break down and rebuild oneself. It brings up all the crap you have ever avoided in your life and plenty you never even knew existed. Then multiply the crap by the number of people on the course and add in their needs and personalities; it was a turbulent time. I saw this as a welcomed, although painful, opportunity to grow, learn and change. Suffice to say, I strapped in for repeated return trips to hell academically, emotionally and practically. I was trying to be the perfect mum and the perfect student. I was hard on myself. Failure was not an option. This was my one and only opportunity to get a degree and nothing was going to get in the way of completing the course, getting a degree and practising as a counsellor. I grabbed the opportunity firmly with both hands and didn't let go, no matter what came my way.

During the final year of my counselling degree, I returned once again to the cancer support centre, this time as a volunteer counsellor. This felt a massive achievement because this is where it had all begun seven years ago. All that had happened, all that I had struggled with, all that had been difficult, all that had nearly destroyed me. Returning as a counsellor to work with cancer patients felt an immense honour. I recognised and understood their struggles because they were so similar to my own. I sat in silence with them as their tears fell because I understood they needed to fall uninterrupted, unrushed and unhushed. It wasn't uncomfortable or difficult to watch. I didn't need to rescue, stop or resolve, because I couldn't. I just needed to be there with them while they spoke of their fears and worries, their losses, their sadness. I had overcome so much to be there. I never lost the sense of compassion working with cancer patients or lost touch with the journey which I had been on, was on and will continue to be on.

It felt very satisfying to return to the cancer support centre as a counsellor and this healed some of the 'trauma' (page 332) cancer had caused. By practising as a counsellor I felt my life had increasing purpose and 'meaning' (page 322), and I was continuing to find a place for cancer.

In October 2012 I graduated with a first class honours degree. I could finally shut away the demons about my academic capability and regrets around higher education. I was capable and I was proud. I took some time out at the end of the course and in January 2013 set up my counselling practice, which has offered me the opportunity to work, but also to balance family life.

> *The degree and career enabled me to complete the 'unfinished business' (page 331) about not having either. Being a counsellor continued to create 'meaning' (page 322) for my life. My 'self-actualisation' (page 331) drove me through the challenging parts of the course because I believed in the goal.*

During this time I received a call from Pete, whose wife Mair had been diagnosed with breast cancer while pregnant with their second baby in 2012. She sadly died when the baby was just three months old. Pete picked my brains about Support for Cancer in Pregnancy, the charity I had set up, as he was in the process of setting up a similar charity called Mummy's Star, in memory of Mair. Pete's passion and drive has seen Mummy's Star develop and thrive, providing valuable support to families who face a diagnosis of cancer during or soon after pregnancy. It has been comforting to see his work and how Mummy's Star makes a difference to the families it supports, as well as raising awareness about cancer during pregnancy and injustices around treatment. With the charity in mind, the profits from book sales of the *Two Faces of Cancer* will be donated to Mummy's Star.

For further information about the charity and the work it does, please take a look at www.mummysstar.org.

Helping other people gives 'meaning' (page 322) to my life and I feel I have such a connection with anyone who is diagnosed with cancer, especially during pregnancy.

CHAPTER 12

"Storms make trees take deeper roots."

Dolly Parton

Hours, days, weeks, months and years passed, sometimes slowly, sometimes quickly, with anniversaries and milestones, good days and not such good days, illnesses and holidays, arguments and differences. My insatiable energy remained; a hunger to achieve, to live, and to avoid my feelings and death. I was constantly driven and never felt satisfied. I called it passion, but it wasn't really; it was avoidance of the fear and anger which I hadn't yet processed.

Life varied from the mundane to the outrageous. Ian and I got married on a beach in Mauritius on my fortieth birthday, holding the girls in our arms. Afterwards we ate chips and olives on the beach and watched the sunset while the girls paddled in the pool in their bridesmaid dresses.

It was gorgeous and posh, and yet so simple and without fuss.

I did school runs, cleared up after stomach bugs, learnt various ways of teaching phonics and re-learnt my times tables. I watched hours of *Peppa Pig,* which morphed into *Hannah Montana,* which morphed into *Take Me Out* and *Gogglebox.* I listened and supported the girls as their problems changed from disagreements around toys, to clothes, make-up, friends, boys, social media feeds, careers and GCSE choices. We chatted about alcohol, swearing, snogging, drugs and periods. Boundaries, bedtimes and relationships changed. The bond and love for them deepened. I was grateful for each day and milestone I got to spend with them. It wasn't always fun or easy, but it was a privilege. I hoped I could be Poppy and Bonnie's mum for just one more day. Just one more day of health and life, please. The cycle of appointments and checks continued, punctuating diary pages, and creating anxious times.

Life was ticking along nicely, my counselling practice building. The girls were settled. Life was good. Life was being lived. Cancer was parked. And then the curveball struck, unexpected, unseen, unheard. *Boom.* In August 2012 I had a sense that the tamoxifen was no longer working. I had no symptoms, just an uneasy hushed sense. In April 2013, when I had my annual mammogram, I was unusually upset during the build-up to the test, breaking down and crying during the appointment. I knew something was wrong, but I didn't know what or where. I remained silent. I had no lumps or bumps, just a niggling intuition which didn't leave, even when the results of the mammogram came back clear. I could not shake off the thudding and permanent tiredness that enveloped me over the summer of 2013, but still no lumps or bumps, no signs or symptoms. Fear circled me, waiting to strike. It was the school holidays and I was tired running the girls around. But cancer tired is a different sort of tiredness, a tiredness that isn't satisfied by rest or sleep. I am now acutely aware of the subtle differences between types of tiredness.

My ten-year check-up was due on Thursday 12th September 2013. Summer was ending and Poppy had just started secondary school. The weekend had been perfect, spending a day with Poppy, browsing art and eating lunch in Brighton. We travelled back, laughing together, with a massive painting wrapped in bubble wrap on the back seat. The weekend ended happy and relaxed.

I began the week conducting the check that my oncologist would be performing on Thursday. No surprises, I would be in control, he wouldn't find anything I didn't know about, a check that I had begun and ended many times. I began feeling along my jaw line, moving the tips of my fingers left and right in parallel at simultaneous speed, then moving downwards to my collar bones, left and right. I then moved to my breasts and armpits. Only this time I didn't get as far as my breasts and armpits, because there, just above my left collar bone, was a lump, a fucking big lump. I knew what it was straight away. Fuck. How long had that been there?

This was the start of my week, finding a lump which, without even having to see a doctor or have a biopsy, I knew was cancer. I now had to wait until Thursday lunchtime to get a medical opinion, information, tests, diagnosis and treatment plan. I asked Ian to feel and see what he thought.

He thought it felt the same as last time. His face turned away. There was no point going to my GP or calling the hospital – with an oncology appointment already booked for four days' time I wasn't going to get seen any earlier. I would have to sit it out. I cried a lot over those few days, the not knowing and yet the so knowing. I was scared. I felt a failure.

My sister offered to come with me to the appointment and, unusually, I accepted. I generally went to appointments on my own, preferring to sit alone with my anxiety rather than engage with banal chit-chat which I found exhausting and irritating rather than distracting. I didn't want to impose my anxiety on others. I just wanted to sit and try and hold it all together. I told the girls what I had found; succinctly, matter of factly, detached from the terror within me. Time, hours, days, minutes passed. And then it was Thursday. Fuck. Fuck. Fuck. I was back in the land of fucking fuck again.

I had been due to see the registrar as this was a routine check-up and consultations with the consultant are at a premium. My oncologist had seen my name on the patient list and had asked to see me, citing that we had known each other a long time and he was going to discharge me today. Today was supposed to be discharge day, the day we would say goodbye. Maybe we would reminisce about the last ten years. I would no doubt say thank you and wish him well, maybe shed a tear or two at what had been achieved and not lost. Little did he know what was about to walk through the door and that it was going to be another hello rather than a goodbye. Hello cancer. Hello chemo. Hello months of treatment. Hello months of recovery. Hello death. Hello fear. Hello depression. Hello scalp. Hello conversations no one wants to have. Hello uncertainty. Goodbye life.

I waited for my name to be called. My breathing was fast and shallow. My name was called and I managed to haul myself from the grey sweaty plastic waiting room chair, inching towards bad news and change. I entered the hot, bright, white room, my life blazing out at the same velocity. I took my place on a seat adjacent to his big table with sprawling papers and a smart pen, the last few breaths and moments before I became a cancer patient once again. We greeted and I held it together as I explained my discovery.

We moved swiftly into the examination room. My sister waited in the consultation room. Paper roll was rolled and I took my horizontal, topless position on the bed. In moments his cool and slightly damp hands were on me. Within seconds the lump was being described as 'suspicious'. He returned to the consultation room to make some enquiries. I was being sent straight away for a blood test and biopsy, and I was to come back next week for the results. I was aware, via Google, of the latest research for this type of recurrence (the CALOR trial), and that chemo would be likely. I was also aware the location of this cancer was not good news regarding my survival.

There was a mixture of relief and fear as I headed along the familiar corridors to the other departments for the tests, relief that some of the not knowing was temporarily abated and fear of what lay ahead. I was also angry about the disruption this was going to have on our lives and my work. I was anxious at the changes that would need to take place to accommodate being treated for cancer.

Just a few minutes later I was being prepped for another core biopsy. This biopsy was equally as unpleasant as the first. There was a lot of positioning and repositioning to be able to take it accurately and safely. It was gruesome to feel someone poking something about inside me and I had to maintain all my focus not to pass out. According to my sister, who came in with me, there was a lot of blood. I left the room feeling bruised, with a large dressing covering the biopsy sites. I then went for a blood test to check my blood for any signs that cancer was elsewhere. I went home dazed but knowing all that could have been done had been done that day. I would now just have to wait until next week for the results and treatment plan.

> *My oncologist's behaviour made this time safe for me. I trusted him, what he said and that he would do everything he could for me, which gave me hope. He created a plan and time frame within which my anxiety could focus and sit; it had an end point. I once again became 'logical' (page 332) and practical to counteract the feelings of fear and anxiety and to feel 'in control' (page 333) and stable in the chaos.*

Following the communication carnage which I experienced back in August 2003 at this stage, I only told a few family and friends about what was potentially going to be happening. It was still difficult to deal with their reactions and I felt guilty about the upset and concern it would cause them. It's hard to know that within a few words, carefully chosen rehearsed and delivered, you are going to change someone's day. One word can change so much in their life.

The change in your life, and the impact it has on theirs. But it had to be done. I was very practical and brief when I told the girls, enough for them to know, not enough for them to worry. They didn't seem overly concerned or troubled. They accepted my words, calmly. Maybe I was calm and detached from my fear and anxiety when I spoke them. Maybe they had no idea or concept to compare with. I made a few phone calls and told everyone else by text. I went to bed tired, with the worry and strain of having held it together and knowing I was going to have to hold it together for a lot longer to keep it safe and stable for the girls.

I was in a void for the week between the biopsy and returning for the results, and decided to keep the commitments I had made as they provided a focus. Ironically I had applied for a job at the cancer support centre and had been invited for an interview the next day. This could be a challenge. I dug deep. I chose an outfit which covered the biopsy site and dressing, pinned, or rather nailed, on a smile and headed for the interview. I was not at my best and didn't get the job. I was a little disappointed as the cancer support centre had meant so much to me, but I also felt that not getting the job was for a reason and something else would come along that would enable me to work with the client group that I identified with.

I had wanted to expand my counselling practice and had booked a coaching course in London, which happened to nestle neatly between the biopsy and results appointments. It was hard to set aside my fears and feelings, but I did to some degree and I emerged two days later with a certificate in executive coaching. I was irritated and distracted every moment I was there and, with the exception of two of the participants, I found everyone else really annoying. I was just in such a different place to them. They were planning coaching careers. I was planning chemo cycles. By the end of the first coffee break they were swapping phone numbers and arranging lifelong friendships. Beam me up and fast-forward to when the certificates of attendance are handed out and get me out of here.

The unknown of the biopsy results was very distracting as I was consumed with trying to keep it all together and stabilise myself; anything which distracted from this irritated me.

I cried and worried a lot over the few days before I returned for the results on Thursday 19th September, ten years and one month to the day since my initial diagnosis. Sadness and anger were part of the process of acceptance. I was grieving for the loss of my lovely life as it was and I didn't want to go back to the hideousness it had been. I was in a good place and didn't want bastard cancer treatment to take that away, not even for a minute. I was also imagining the worst possible cancer scenarios, how far the cancer had spread and how long I had left to live.

My oncologist gave me the results quickly and succinctly. I appreciated his calmness and honesty. I understood what he was saying. I knew where I was and what needed to happen. The pathology report of the biopsy showed it was a similar cancer to previously. The cancer would have been present the first time around, but had lain dormant, silent, lurking in the supraclavicular fossa until now, ten years later, just as my oncologist was going to say goodbye, you are now so low risk you can go, enjoy your life. But of course cancer doesn't follow the script. It does its own thing, silently and unnoticed, until it's multiplying, created the protruding lump rising up from the collar bone.

The cancer was a grade 2 (more aggressive than last time) invasive ductal carcinoma, which was less strongly oestrogen receptive, but now progesterone receptive; the same cancer but different. It had tweaked itself so it could avoid the halting action of the tamoxifen. It had found a way. It found a way to grow again while I was busy bringing up my girls and creating bucket lists and buying art in Brighton.

The treatment plan was outlined and then consented to. Initially there would be four cycles of chemo (but maybe more) followed by radiotherapy. The chemo regime would be docetaxel again, along with another drug called cyclophosphamide, which was one of the drugs from the AC combo from last time. Memories of anxiety and agitation came flooding back when I heard the word docetaxel and I was prescribed lorazepam to take the edge off of this. The fact there was no surgery alarmed me. Just cut the mother fucker bastard out I wanted to say. Tamoxifen was out and letrozole was in, and I would probably be having goserelin as well if the chemo didn't put me into a menopause.

As this information was being given, I mentally went through the pages of my diary to recall what had been planned and what was going to need to be changed. Potentially everything. Work, kids and four big things that I had been looking forward to and planning for a while:

Bonnie's birthday bonanza, a trip to Switzerland, Ian's fiftieth and a trip to Sydney in February 2014. I really didn't want to miss a moment of these, but for now I was going to have to see how things panned out. Would I be up for those things? Actually, would I be alive for those things?

It seemed a lot to ask that the tumour would shrink, let alone disappear, in four chemo sessions and this created further anxiety in me because my oncologist had said that for the radiotherapy to have the best effect, the tumour needed to be as small as possible. The chemo had to work and it had to work well. I'm not too good at failing and anything less than total obliteration of the silent assassin could feel like failure, an epic failure for which I would pay with my life. The pressure felt instantly turned up to full. I mumbled out loud the bargaining taking place in my mind that if this was it, at least I had had a great ten years. My oncologist replied that if we could 'melt this down' there was no reason why I couldn't have another ten years. The blood test had come back normal and my oncologist didn't think that the cancer had spread further than the supraclavicular fossa but he couldn't be certain and I was referred for bone and CT scans to check that this 'wasn't just the tip of an iceberg'. The bad news was being drip fed, one potential disaster at a time.

Please could this be all the bad news for now? Please can the cancer not have spread anywhere else? I had children to bring up and a bucket list to finish. He then went on to say that the results of these scans would need to be given face-to-face, so I could be supported if the cancer had spread further than the supraclavicular fossa site.

My 'be perfect' (page 329) and 'try harder' (page 329)

drivers were in evidence at this stage. I couldn't bear the thought of failing at chemo. I hadn't been good enough not to get cancer again. I hadn't tried hard enough not to get cancer again and so I couldn't fail at chemo. To counteract these feelings I tried to be the perfect patient by turning up smiling and happy, attending every appointment and taking every tablet. I felt that if I was perfect I could avoid death itself. I was also 'bargaining' (page 326) that if I was going to die, I had had a great ten years and had been the best mum I could to Poppy and Bonnie.

I appreciated the way my oncologist told me the tests required and their implications to me in parts, which gave me time to process each one before the next one was delivered. This felt manageable, emotionally, because I could process each 'trauma' (page 332) before the next one arrived. However, I was desperate to know the whole story as the unknown caused me anxiety. I was 'angry' (page 326) at the cancer for taking away what I loved, and had worked so hard to achieve, while I had the treatment and recovered, and that I was going to lose the 'meaning' (page 322) from my life once more. I was about to be returned to 'stage 1' (page 317) where the world felt unsure and unsafe because my life was under threat again. It felt good to know about the treatment plan which created safety and hope for me.

I left the hospital knowing the lump was cancer, but with new anxieties focusing on how far the cancer had spread and feeling under pressure for the treatment to work. It was my responsibility to make sure it worked. It was my life that would be ending if it didn't. What if? What if? What if? I didn't want to say goodbye to my girls, not now, not as we were hitting the teenage years. There was so much more to see and do. They needed me. I needed them. I left with the information and treatment plan, which I needed to get my head round and communicate to the people in my life. I now had to wait for the next set of test appointments and results to get the whole ghastly picture. Today, as it turned out, was just a headline. There were now so many bigger questions that needed answering.

CHAPTER 13

"New beginnings are often disguised as painful endings."

Lao Tzu

Waiting for the CT and bone scan appointments was a nervous and anxious time. My mind was constantly busy; I wanted to scream and shout to exorcise the thoughts, feelings and internal trauma, the constant 'what ifs?' The appointments would lead to the tests and the tests to the results. I wanted the results, but I also didn't. I didn't want any more bad news or difficult conversations. It was unbearable at times not to know how far the cancer had spread, if it had spread. I was at my limit and felt, at times, that my head would explode under the pressure. I was glad at this point that I had reduced the amount of information I was giving out. I only had my thoughts and feelings to manage, and that was enough, not the tears and fears of others joining them.

The CT scan (a CT scan is a scan of your body which produces detailed pictures using X-rays – the scan is taken while you lie flat on a bed with a cylindrical scanner like a giant ring doughnut passing around you) was to see if the cancer had spread to my liver and/or lungs, in which case I would be terminally ill. I had booked another training course, but when the scan date appointment came, it was on the same day so I cancelled the course. I needed to be realistic and prioritise. I was beginning to recognise that it was okay to say I needed help or I couldn't do or achieve something because I needed to do something else.

I was beginning to learn it was okay not to 'be perfect' (page 329) or 'be strong' (page 329) all of the time, and this reduced my stress and anxiety levels.

I had not had a CT scan before, so this was all new and therefore, initially, the anxiety centred around the procedure rather than the outcome. I was having a scan 'with contrast' which required me not to eat for four hours prior to the scan, four whole hours without food. Not eating is quite torturous for me as I could quite easily spend all day, every day, eating. I arrived at the hospital and waited, and was then asked to drink a litre of water over an hour before the scan. I waited and weed and carried on drinking and waiting and weeing. I was already bored of drinking, waiting and weeing.

My named was called. The procedure was explained. I stripped off and gowned up, carrying my possessions in an old bashed-up supermarket shopping basket. I looked like a vagrant. I got onto the scanning bed and had an IV needle inserted into a vein in my arm. The nurse explained what to expect when a shot of iodine was administered: a metallic taste in my mouth, a hot flush through my body and that I would feel like I was wetting myself but I wouldn't. Sounded lots of fun.

The nurses silently retreated behind a sealed, glazed, partitioned section of the room and further communications were made via an intercom. The giant doughnut scanner began rotating, gathering speed and whirring around my body. I lay as still as I could on the stationary bed. The giant doughnut was measuring, detecting and comparing health and illness. Looking at my vital organs; what should be there and what shouldn't. Instructions to breathe or not breathe were delivered via the intercom, as was the warning that the iodine was on its way. I felt like I was part of a scene in a sci-fi film. The IV drip clicked into action and a shot of iodine was administered remotely, disappearing into my arm. As it surged around my body I experienced all of the previously mentioned bodily sensations. It really did feel like I was wetting myself. I felt compelled to check the bed when the scans had finished and the IV was removed – I hadn't.

Once the scan was finished, my anxiety instantly focused on the unknown of the test results, I was in a permanent state of stress and distress until I knew if the cancer had spread.

The bone scan was booked for the day after the CT scan. It was a stressful week but not as stressful as getting the results, I bargained to myself. I went back to hospital number two for the bone scan. Another walk along endless, soulless corridors, jammed-up car parks and confusing signs. I am mobile and capable, and can only imagine the assistance needed by someone less so. Life as a cancer patient was turning into a full-time job. There was not just the stress from having the scan, but worrying about getting to the appointment on time, the availability of a parking space at the hospital, whether the children were okay, whether I would be back in time for the school pick up, what we should have for dinner. Maybe I should worry less about those; maybe they are a diversion to avoid thinking about the seriousness of the situation.

I headed to nuclear medicine. The usual checks were made with a double dose of questioning regarding pregnancy status. No, I wasn't pregnant. I definitely wasn't pregnant. I wasn't going to be pregnant any time soon; in fact I wasn't going to be pregnant ever again. Cancer had fucked that up for me. Barren and infertile. Once we had that sorted, the nice man gloved and gowned up and injected a mysterious liquid from a lead container into me. The routine was as before. Bugger off, drink loads of water and come back for the bone scan four hours later.

I headed off to drink more water than I thought was possible. I met up with a friend for a very posh and fabulous lunch in a local town, before I returned for another battle of the car parking spaces, the endless, soulless corridors and the scan. The scan was painless and simple. I was merely required to lay motionless while strapped to a bed, wondering about my life and what the fuck was going on inside of me. I could hear my stomach gurgling from lunch. The bone scan machine passed silently over me, detecting any menacing gathering of the radioactive isotope which would indicate a spread of the breast cancer to my bones. Someone somewhere was now looking at the images of my body. Someone somewhere knew if cancer was growing, symptomless, elsewhere in my body or not. But that wasn't yet me.

The moment the scan had finished I was anxious to get back to pick the girls up from school, craving routine and normality to counterbalance the uncertainty. I was quick off the bed, said my thank yous and goodbyes, and power-walked back along the endless, soulless corridors to the packed car park, back to fresh air and back to my life. To see Poppy and Bonnie come out of their classrooms, to hear about their day, was vital to keeping me going; normality, me doing the job I had signed up for, being a mum, being there, not dying before I had completed that job. There wasn't room for cancer in that.

I now had to wait for the results of these scans. It felt as if my whole life was on a cliff edge. I could fall at any moment, physically or emotionally. The results would determine which of two very different paths I would be travelling along: the path of death, coffin selection and a funeral, or the path of more time, another Christmas and another bucket list. I tried to keep busy, reminding myself that my incessant worrying was not going to change what was or was not going on in my body. Those few days and weeks were tough, as autumn took away summer and cancer took away my life's meaning.

I was extremely anxious during this time about the scan results and the enormity of the impact they would have on my life. I now had to sit with the uncertainty of the unknown until I got the results.

There is a lot of waiting when you are being treated for cancer, and then some more waiting, followed by even more waiting and then after that, you wait some more. Waiting for things to grow or shrink, waiting for treatments, waiting for tests, waiting for results, waiting for appointments, waiting for phone calls, waiting for time to pass, waiting for a bag of meds to take home. Waiting should come with a warning sign; it can cause frustration and, as the frustration builds, it wants to burst out at something or someone possibly not even connected with waiting. On top of the waiting there is plenty of unknown. The unknown follows a similar trajectory and outcome as waiting.

I was used to my life running to time and to plan, which created feelings of safety in the unknown future and vastness of time. Cancer took me away from my 'freedom' (page 322) to choose and plan into the unknown, which created feelings of being 'out of control' (page 333), which created anxiety.

The day arrived when I was going to find out the results of the CT and bone scan, the day I would find out if I was going to live or die. I still have flashbacks when I wear the top I wore that day, a pretty swirling paisley pattern, calming tones and hues of blue. I had managed to contain the anxiety in the build-up to the day by distracting myself, but as the day dawned I was totally terrified. Ian came with me and we made our way back to the third hospital, beginning another car park place scramble and another wait on sweaty grey plastic chairs.

The clinic was very busy, and hot. I sweated in my pretty patterned top. I could feel my heart pounding rhythmically like an orchestral drum. *Boom, boom, boom, boom.* I sat nervously waiting for my name to be called, hoping and searching each time a medic appeared in the waiting room to see if it was my oncologist. After what seemed like an eternity of sweating and pounding of anxiety and fear, my name was called. But it was by a doctor I had never met. This moment felt totally unbearable; I just wanted to be in the safe care of my oncologist who I trusted. If I was going to be diagnosed with secondary cancer, secondary cancer which was going to kill me, I wanted to be hearing it from his voice. But it doesn't work like that. Hundreds of doctors, and thousands of patients; I was just one of many on that day in that clinic.

I slowed my pace as I walked into the examination room. I was frantically searching and scanning for my oncologist to see if he was there, to see if I could create a diversion, and a reason to be seen by him. He wasn't. I swiftly switched to plan B. How could I quickly establish a relationship with someone I had never met and then be told potentially life-changing news? I have realised that unlike the counselling world where the work is built on and through a relationship, the medical world isn't. The medical world is about a symptom, a diagnosis, a treatment and with any luck, a recovery. A scan here, a scan there, no one cared. No one had the time to care about my life-changing news. It didn't matter to them who told me or how they told me.

We exchanged polite hellos and handshakes, and in the momentary space of his hesitation I said I was there to get the results of the scans. He looked blank and shuffled a few papers. The results of the scans were not there. I didn't think it was possible, but during those seconds my anxiety and heart rate increased further. The orchestral drums were now playing through a festival-style speaker, loudly. New doctor tried to access the results via the computer, but was unable to as the scans were taken at hospitals one and two, and I was now at hospital three. Hospital three had no computer links to one and two. Hospitals one and two were less than thirty miles away, but may as well have been in another galaxy at this moment in time.

I wanted to be sick. I had held my fears and I had held my anxiety for so long, I now couldn't hold on any more. I needed to know. New doctor seemed to sense this and said he would phone someone. New doctor's friend was able to access the bone scan results and to confirm that this particular scan was clear and that the cancer hadn't spread to my bones. He communicated this by making a thumbs-ups sign while he concluded the phone call, a gesture of universal meaning. I felt that the impending heart attack that I was experiencing had been narrowly averted. He was unable to access the CT scan results, but was 90% sure that with the bone scan being clear, there would be no spread to my liver or lungs. My breathing began to return to normal, slowly slowing as danger and fear passed. Some news was better than no news. After examining and measuring the tumour, he upped his estimate to 95%. I could breathe again. My heart rate and anxiety continued to subside. The meeting concluded with him advising me to paint my nails with nail varnish, because daylight interacting with my nails could cause them to fall off while I was receiving the chemo. Oh well, if nothing else, at least my nails would look good over the coming months, while everything else fell apart.

We went and had a coffee (I had an enormous piece of carrot cake too) and a walk in the warm autumn sunshine, before coming back for a pre-chemo appointment which was scheduled for later in the day. The daylight and fresh air felt good, and was a welcome but temporary distraction from the hideousness of it all.

There was little time to process the scan results before the next tranche of information was being presented. The next wait was shorter, in fact non-existent; they were waiting for us. That was a first. We met with one of the nurses from the chemo suite to run through the chemo treatment. As the nurse began explaining the potential side effects of chemo, the horror of the side effects I had experienced last time jumped to the forefront of my mind from a filed-away past I hoped I'd never have to experience again, ever. But cancer isn't like that, it lingers and lurks and returns. I didn't really hear the rest of what she was saying. My mind was saturated with flashbacks and became closed off to further information. I disengaged to keep safe.

In less than sixty hours my life was going to change. I was officially going to be returning to the role of a cancer patient, where this becomes the role that defines you, not your job or your achievements or your hobbies. A cancer patient, where everything else falls after or around this role or is affected or influenced by it. I made the most of the weekend, counting down the hours until the drugs and the treatment began. I tucked away the bag of drugs that I had been sent home with until the last possible moment. The dread of treatment was now just hours away.

CHAPTER 14

"Let your hopes, not your hurts, shape your future."

Robert H. Schuller

I rose early on Monday 7th October ahead of chemo cycle one, relishing the last few hours before the drugs went in. I put on my running shoes for what I knew would be the last time in a while. I savoured the run, the freedom, the fresh air, the autumn light and the berried hedgerows. I came back and took the steroids, had breakfast and got ready for the day ahead. I did the school run, happy and smiley as if none of it mattered, as if I was heading off for a normal day instead of the chemo unit. I went and bought a posh picnic lunch, as if to treat myself during the day ahead. I then took the lorazepam and waited for my sister to collect me (driving on that amount of drugs was going to be a no-no). As the lorazepam began to work, a feeling of giddiness crept through my body. Unstable. Slightly sick. Woozy. Wobbly. My sister arrived and I got in the car. I was in a foggy drug-infused state and these were only the pre-chemo drugs.

The chemo clinic had grown since my last visit and was now in a day unit attached to a cancer ward, instead of small rooms in a basement. The rooms were light and airy and hot. The heating goes on at a certain time of the year and stays on with no regard to weather or the temperature outside. I smiled at patients as I passed by, silently thinking 'I know what you have been through'. We wove our way through the ward to the day unit. Each face I passed was on its own journey. Each face had received its own diagnosis. Each face was a façade for thoughts and feelings, each face hiding struggles and side effects, hopes and fears. Each face had a pathology and treatment plan as individual as the face it belonged to. Each face had been assigned a unique cocktail of drugs with unpronounceable names. Each face had faces in their lives who were as frightened as them.

We arrived at the check-in desk, which is not as exciting as an airport check-in; I had no choice but to attend and destination health was not guaranteed. The familiar 'Are you the right person?' checks began. I was shown to a seat and waited, feeling increasingly woozy as the steroids and lorazepam circulated my body.

A nurse and a tray of drugs arrived. Each drug carefully named, dated and labelled. This was tough. I'd normally ponder for hours about taking a couple of paracetamol, so all these drugs went against my personal choices, but with cancer there is no choice. The checks were made again and a cannula (a small tube which is inserted into a vein via a needle to administer medicine) was inserted and fixed in place with a large white dressing. Saline was flushed in to check the cannula was correctly positioned. The cold cap was then placed on my head and the straps pulled down under my chin and adjusted until there was the familiar tight fit. A thumping headache joined the woozy feelings. I was kitted up and good to go for chemo. My head began chilling and I became grateful for the hot room as the chill crept through my body.

The cannula became the gateway for drugs and treatment, for health and life. First in was the anti-sickness meds. I was already feeling sick (some chemo drugs trigger chemicals that send signals between nerves, which in turn created a feeling of nausea, and the anti-sickness meds block these signals) and I hadn't even had anything that was going to make me sick yet. Next in was the first chemo drug, cyclophosphamide which was given by injection. The clear liquid left the syringe and entered my body, silently. Kill that fucker, I thought. There was no going back now. This was followed by the docetaxel, which was given by infusion over a couple of hours. A further dose of steroids followed in tablet form, a full-on day out of drugs.

I began to look paler and greener by the second. I tried to keep my head as still as possible and any movements to a minimum. A lunch trolley loaded with sandwiches and red jellies circulated. I feebly waved it past so as not to add to the waves of nausea. My posh picnic went uneaten.

My sister sat and waited with me. Texts were sent and received throughout the day. Social media updates made and glanced at. I could keep in touch with my lovely life as the drugs entered and circulated and my hair follicles were protected by the head chilling. Drugs dripped in and time passed by. I was so green and nauseous by the end of the treatment that I stayed in hospital for an extra couple of hours before I felt well enough to leave, clutching a grey disposable cardboard sick bowl just in case. There was the obligatory party bag of drugs to be taken over the next few days to recover from this cycle of chemo and prepare for the next. I have no recollection of the rush hour journey home. I felt foggy and woozy. I hoped I could remember which drugs to take when and how to administer the course of injections that would begin in a couple of days.

That night there were further anti-sickness meds to take. My body was screaming no. It was full enough of drugs. I felt I had taken a lifetime's worth in one day. Dinner, children, sleep. The grey disposable cardboard sick bowl never far from sight or reach. I woke the next day still feeling foggy and woozy, and began the day with the final doses of the steroids and further anti-sickness meds and a large glass of pure, clear water to cleanse the cocktails of drugs and poison I felt I had taken.

The anti-sickness meds were prescribed for the following week, but of course I wouldn't be needing them. I would be over this in a couple of days, and back to my usual bouncing self. Busy, busy, busy; health, vitality, energy, focus. But I wasn't. I felt shit, physically and emotionally. I learnt through chucking up several times, including in Marks and Spencer's food hall, to take the anti-sickness meds with regularity and longevity, just like the doctor had said. Eating also helped alleviate the nausea. In fact I'd crave carbs and fatty foods. I mean, who doesn't love a Marks and Spencer's sausage roll or twenty? Thousands of calories consumed daily. I was constantly hungry and constantly eating. I began piling on the pounds. I put on two stone over the coming months, which I assumed, based on cancer treatment number one, would fall off easily when I returned to life. I was wrong; it was ruddy hard to shift. What I didn't know then was that, because I was ten years older, the treatment was aimed at reducing as many hormones as possible, making me as menopausal as possible; therefore weight gain was easy and weight loss was difficult.

The physical feelings varied from the 2003 chemo cycles, where week one had been okay and week two awful. I expected and planned for the same this time. It wasn't. It was reversed, with week one being awful and week two okay. The sickness and nausea on day four was so terrible I could hardly move and I upgraded from the grey hospital freebie to a large red plastic bucket positioned on a large blue plastic mat placed below my head on the sofa, just in case. Everything, even water, tasted disgusting and I would drink it through a straw placed as far back in my mouth as possible so I didn't taste it. Drinking plenty of fluids was important to flush out the toxicity of the drugs from my blood, liver and urinary tract so that I didn't end up with infections.

It was an unpleasant but necessary time. I allowed time and space for the chemo to do its job and for me to heal. It was a very simple existence and one which felt right. My priorities changed. I wanted to be there for the girls, to keep our lives as normal as possible, so the crazy nights out, the giggling girly lunches and long dog walks ceased. I conserved my energy to be the best possible parent I could. The TV was on and I just lay around, changing sofas and channels periodically, watching the sun, clouds, leaves, birds and winter vistas passing by. This was no doubt what my body needed but my mind hovered just above depression. The trainers gathered dust. I could barely walk to the car I felt so knackered. It was hard letting go of the things I loved, but I knew I had to do my part and let my body rest and recuperate.

This time around I had 'acceptance' (page 327) of what needed to happen in the short term to have the greatest chance of having time with my children in the longer term. I was able to accept the change in the 'meaning' (page 322) of my life for this period with less struggle and 'anger' (page 326) because I trusted that my 'freedom' (page 322) to choose would return in the future.

The docetaxel element of the chemo regime was known to cause neutropenic sepsis (a potentially life-threatening condition where a type of white blood cell that defends the body against bacterial and fungal infections becomes dangerously low), as it had with the chemo in 2003. Fast-forward ten years and now G-CSF (a drug which kick-starts the bone marrow into producing the white blood cells that the chemo has knocked off along with the cancer cells), which prevents neutropenic sepsis, is given routinely. I would need to start the five-day course of injections on day three of the chemo cycle.

The injections could be given by a district nurse, but my guilt was accumulating at the amount of NHS resources I was using, so I said I would administer the injections myself. It was now day three of the chemo cycle and I needed to have the first of five G-CSF injections for this cycle. If only I could remember how to do them. The demo had been made post-steroid, post-lorazepam, and post-chemo, when all I could do was focus on was not being sick.

I'm not one for any medical procedure and, as I was about to discover, especially one that I was going to self-administer via a needle. Out came the box of G-CSF with a sheet of instructions the size of a small dining table. The previous Caesareans were going to be useful at this point as there was a thick wad of flesh which had no feeling, perfect for inserting a needle. Children gathered to watch with faces of macabre curiosity. A friend made sense of the instructions and supervised the mixing and shaking of the vials, and the drawing up of the contents into a syringe.

With the count of one, two, three and a deep breath, I put the needle into my stomach only not quite as deftly as you see on TV medical shows. Breathe. I was okay, I was still alive, I hadn't hit an artery, and I wasn't bleeding out. Breathe. All I had to do was push the plunger in and I was good to go. It quickly became another matter, actually pressing the plunger into my flesh. I didn't think that I could. There was no other way forward. I had to push the plunger and yet hold the needle stable and vertically in me. This was grim. How hard should I push? Would the needle snap off inside me? I felt faint and nauseous, but I did it.

By the third G-CSF injection of each chemo cycle, the side effects began. My bones started to throb like a muscle spasm and ache like flu. On the first cycle it was so intense I thought I had broken my back and that the bone scan was wrong and I had cancer in my spine. A quick midnight visit to Google confirmed this was incorrect and it was the side effects of the G-CSF injections. A couple of doses of paracetamol improved things.

And a new cycle of life emerged. Chemo on a Monday, felt okayish Tuesday, Wednesday I began to feel ill, and Thursday was a write off, followed by moments on Friday, Saturday and Sunday where I did begin to feel lively. By the following Tuesday, and eight days post-chemo, I felt able to function but I was very careful to rest and not overdo anything. My purpose was to have the treatment and give myself the best chance of survival and be there for my girls. If that meant doing not much, then that is what I would need to do.

If I held onto the temporality of the revised 'meaning' (page 322) of my life, I could manage my thoughts and feelings for the majority of the time. Once the chemo cycles were in place this provided safety with its structure. It was hard at times with my 'hurry up' (page 330) driver wanting to achieve so much and yet having to sit back and watch time pass by unproductively.

The constant touching of the tumour began the week after chemo. Searching, hoping, checking. Had it gone? Had it changed? Had it got smaller? Searching for a sign; I prodded and poked myself all the time. I prodded and poked myself so much I couldn't remember what the tumour felt like in the first place. I had discomfort in my neck muscles for months after from this. Week 1, no change. Week 2, no change, fuck I was in trouble. Die you bastard. Week 3, the tumour felt softer but not smaller.

I was desperately hoping for the tumour to be smaller, which would alleviate my feelings of anxiety about 'death' (page 321) and being 'out of control' (page 333) of the treatment and the effect it would have on the cancer.

Bonnie's tenth birthday fell just seven days after chemo cycle one on Monday 14th October. Part of the three-day birthday festival was going to have to take part without me. I didn't want to risk picking up an infection by being in contact with a group of ten-year-olds. A good friend stepped in and took my place. She made a cake and helped Ian run the party at a local venue. For the family party the following day, I relinquished the need to be a flawless hostess with homemade dishes planned and served with precision and perfection. I asked guests to bring a dish each. It was lovely and also liberating not having the stress and responsibility to be perfect. It wasn't what I planned, but I was beginning to learn that things didn't have to look as I had planned in my head. They could be just as good if they just evolved without a plan.

It was actually a great relief not to be functioning from my 'be perfect' driver (page 329) and to let people help me.

I headed for the pre-chemo cycle number two appointment on my own and two days earlier than the hospital wanted. Lovely Brother was over from Sydney on a course in

Switzerland and we had booked a weekend months beforehand to go over and see him. There was no way I was missing that. There was no way cancer was taking that from me. There were lots of concerns, but the medical one centred around having the routine pre-chemo blood test early, as it may show that my immune system was not well enough recovered to receive the next cycle of chemo, in which case it would be delayed. I was willing to take that chance. Any fallout could be sorted but I wasn't missing out on my trip.

My name was called and I was pleased to see the doctor that I had seen last time, a brief moment of stability. He had a letter in front of him and said he now had the results of the CT and bone scans, which had not been available last time. I looked down and saw a white page containing a long numbered list on the paper. Fuck, the cancer was everywhere, I was now going to hear, what I had tried so hard to avoid for so long. In that spilt second I wanted to feel in control and said 'It's everywhere isn't it?' Somehow, if I said the words it would be less of a shock, and momentarily I would be in control. He looked up at me shocked and confused, and said 'no' and that the scans were clear and the cancer was only in the supraclavicular fossa. I took an enormous breath. Relief. Reprieve. Breathe. He then examined me, agreeing the tumour felt softer. This was positive, and the reassurance I was craving so desperately. I was heading in the right direction. I was doing something right. I reported back about the nausea and he added in an extra anti-sickness drug and suggested I ate or drank something with ginger in. I hate anything ginger, so that wouldn't be happening. I left with an excited heart and a bag of prescription drugs and I began to think about setting off to Switzerland, a weekend of chemo reprieve, a welcome distraction in the cancer chaos.

With kids and pets cared for, Ian and I headed off via car, plane and train to Lake Lucerne. Switzerland was breathtakingly beautiful, peaceful and calm. We sat drinking coffee in the tranquil autumn sunshine watching exquisitely dressed people walk along the lakeside paths. I was delighted to see my brother; so much had happened since we last met, just over two months ago. We sat wrapped in blankets on a terraced veranda drinking cocktails, Lake Lucerne below us and the mountains behind. I felt out of place in this picturesque setting, with my body concealing its grotesque diagnosis. Who would know? I looked so normal. We spent two days breathing the cleanest, freshest air. I gorged on the air and freedom while I could. We ate fondue in a noisy restaurant, talking and laughing, with cheese dripping everywhere. We took a ferry across from Lucerne to Evian on the other side of the lake and wandered the quaint, cobbled streets and boutique shops. We looked down on the city at night from a church, watching the lights twinkling below us. Cancer and chemo seemed another lifetime away and yet they consumed and distracted me, my mind switching between my two lives.

It felt wonderful to connect with the 'social' (page 323) and 'personal' (page 324) dimensions of my life.

The hair loss started on the flight out. I stood up and looked down – there was a wad of my hair on the headrest. I felt embarrassed and brushed it off. First a few hairs, and then handfuls. I couldn't stop running my fingers through it to check the process, checking the rate of loss and what remained. Hair, my hair, my precious hair was everywhere I had been and I felt like Hansel and Gretel leaving a trail wherever I went. It had begun, the process of change, and there would be no hiding or disguising my role now. Cancer patient. Obvious for all to see, stare at and gawp at; to pity, to think 'thank fuck that's not me'.

Sunday arrived all too soon and our return flight, booked long before the scheduling of the second cycle of chemo, was for late in the evening. I began the day with a large dose of steroids in preparation for the chemo cycle which would begin the next day. The colour began to fade from my face as they took effect. As the weekend had progressed, a huge storm was being predicted to hit the UK in the evening. I was becomingly increasingly worried that our late night flight was going to be cancelled. I didn't want to risk a chemo delay and the implications of a trip that maybe I shouldn't have taken. We changed our tickets to an earlier flight and it was with sadness that we said our goodbyes to Lovely Brother, after a late breakfast and final lakeside walk in the crisp mountain air. Tomorrow was getting nearer and nearer. Tomorrow was defined by a cycle of chemo; chemo cycle number two, chemo cycle number two of four. I was always counting towards or away from something.

As we hugged on the train platform, I wondered if I would ever see Lovely Brother again. Would I survive the remaining three cycles of chemo? Would the chemo work? Was this the final goodbye? The goodbye we don't know is a goodbye? The goodbye that would be okay as we had had a great weekend? I didn't know. I could only hope this wouldn't be.

We made it back safely and on time. The storm arrived after we got back; it was violent and long. The house shook all night. The day began with more steroids and tranquillisers taken with green tea, the polarities of my life, poison and purity. The second cycle of chemo was during half-term, on Monday 28th October, so Ian and the girls accompanied me. I wanted them to witness me as a chemo patient, to alleviate the unknown, to see the whole cycle: the unseen first part; drugs in; the cause of their pale and knackered mum, lying on the sofa, moody and moulting. They seemed keen.

We were unsure if there would be any delays due to fallen debris caused by the storm, so we left a bit earlier, with the steroids and tranquilisers taking effect as we drove. We arrived at the ward. It all felt normal. How could I even consider this as normal? They dropped me off, gazing round and round the room to make sense of this new world, the world of cancer treatment. They settled me in and left. They enjoyed a few hours shopping and, I suspect, drank Coke and ate chips in some burger outlet, while I received drugs in various formats and combinations. They collected me later, woozy and weak. They smelt of hot fat. I smelt of hospital. Their cheeks rosy, mine pale. Their mouths smiling, mine trying not to be sick.

And so the days of taking the right medicine at the right time and on the right days began again, as did the prodding, searching and hoping for a change, and feeling ill and pointless. The tumour felt changed right before the next chemo, in the nick of time. Once I could detect change, I could relax and feel hopeful and safe, if only momentarily. If there was change, I could feel I had tried my hardest. I had done nothing really. I had played a passive role. I was merely the receptacle for cancer and treatment. The cancer would either respond or it wouldn't.

During this time it was Ian's fiftieth birthday. I love a party, but Ian doesn't, so I had to think carefully about what to do, a way to celebrate but not go over the top (that could be a challenge for me). I had booked the outlines of a party early in 2013 but cancelled it because I thought it was not something Ian would like. It turned out it was just as well because Ian's fiftieth fell just before chemo cycle number three. Some friends had been to a lighthouse on the south coast for their wedding anniversary and it seemed like the perfect venue to hire for Ian's birthday; stunning, exclusive and unique. I was able to book the whole lighthouse, six rooms and twelve people. This seemed a good compromise, celebrating but in a low-key way. We managed to keep the whole event a surprise for him. I felt guilty that chemo played a part of both his fortieth and fiftieth birthday celebrations.

Ian had no idea about the weekend and was getting more and more stressed as we drove further and further away from home, and along smaller and smaller roads, until we turned off onto a track. I was giggling more and more the closer we got. His face was a picture when we arrived and our friends jumped out from behind their parked cars. And for a few brief hours the world seemed good and normal, peaceful. We sat drinking champagne in the lighthouse lantern room, watching the sunset over the sea. Laughing and reminiscing, until the steroids came out again on Sunday morning. Chemo cycle number three was on the horizon. We packed up our stuff, hugged and said our goodbyes, heading home knowing what would take place in less than twenty-four hours' time.

My oncologist had seen and acknowledged me in the waiting room for the pre-chemo appointment, but my name was called by a young doctor who I hadn't met before. Anxiety up. I found the constant cycle of new doctors stressful. I didn't know, or therefore, trust them with saving my life. I wanted some confirmation that tumour change was happening and as he hadn't met me or felt the tumour before, I was not confident this would take place. He had nothing to compare it against, only what was written in my now bulging case notes. I wanted to ask what he thought, but knew it was pointless. Instead I began to ask him increasingly difficult and awkward questions to vent my frustration. I could see his discomfort and yet I continued being childish at not getting what I wanted. I saw his weakness and asserted my power. It was unkind of me and I'm not proud of that behaviour, but fear and frustration take us away from the people we are. My oncologist had heard me with the young doctor and came into the room, maybe to rescue him. I felt an instant relief and reassurance seeing him. He calmed me. He felt the tumour and said he could feel change. Relief and reassurance began soothing my fear and frustration. I felt topped up and motivated to keep going, to keep trying.

The only person who I trusted in all of this was my oncologist. No one else filled me with feelings of safety. This goes to show the strength of feelings involved and the impact that feelings of trust and safety can have on us, especially in times of threat and trauma.

As the treatment progressed, my appearance changed. My hair thinned, my waistline thickened, dark circles developed under my eyes. I looked ill. Pale. Devoid of energy. Just surviving. Hibernating. Actually I looked fucking awful. Health and life drifting away. I was morphing by the day, hour, minute. My body was being battered by the treatment. The assassin was being taken out, slowly, surely, repeatedly.

Inactivity didn't suit me physically or mentally. I was sad and felt pathetic that my life was reduced to lying on the sofa for days at a time, eating the weirdest of food combinations, watching time and life passing me by, frustrated at this waste of time. Day four of the cycle became the day I felt physically the most ill and day five was when the mental pain and sadness hit. When the boredom arrived, I knew I was feeling better. My energy and focus could venture further than my ill, fat body and the TV remote.

A friend accompanied me to chemo cycle number three; she was caring and kind and we giggled quietly in the corner as the drugs arrived and were administered. She would come round and just sit with me and we would watch rubbish daytime TV. I was capable of little more than breathing in the weak winter light. The drugs, the winter darkness, the injections, the appointments, the monotony continued.

The fourth, and potentially final, pre-chemo check was made by yet another doctor. My heart fell as my familiar name was called by an unfamiliar voice and face. I just wanted to see my oncologist and feel safe. The latest new doctor was unsure and hesitant in his manner, which rocked me further. I needed a stable and secure base amidst the unknown and uncertainty. I needed someone confident to take the lead, to hold me in my anxiety and fear against the silent and deadly assassin living within. I was frustrated at not seeing my oncologist and began asking the new doctor questions about how he would know if four cycles of chemo had been enough. The Christmas break was imminent and I was aware the clinics would not run, and I didn't want to be lost in the system and not have further chemo if I needed it. I needed to know what the plan was. I needed to counteract the unknown and the uncertainty. I pushed and pushed with my questions. A monstrous brat became unleashed in the room, determined to have what she wanted, the stress and anxiety at the unknown contained no more. I was now fighting for what I needed with no regards for hospital protocol or how I was behaving.

I would feel guilty after behaving like this, but the need to know and feel 'in control' (page 333) overrode my values and boundaries. At times I played the role of 'persecutor' (page 328) to have my needs met.

I had taken my oncologist some of his favourite chocolate and a Christmas card and gave them to a nurse to pass on to him. I wasn't expecting to see him but wanted to say thank you for all he had done for me again. To my utter delight he came into the consultation room mid-appointment to say hello and thank you. My rock was there, my safety vessel; I felt calm and safe, my monster tamed and I reverted to my dignified self in his presence. It was in this moment I realised my attachment to my oncologist and wondered how healthy it was. If I couldn't manage this without him, what would happen when he left or retired? I realised I needed to work on this, but not now, now I just needed to know he was there. He felt the tumour and commented on its continued shrinkage and okayed a CT scan to identify if further chemo would be needed.

I recognised I had formed a slightly unhealthy 'insecure attachment' (page 317) to my oncologist because he was not always available. I realised how safe he made the world, as per 'stage 1' (page 317), in this foreign and unsafe land of cancer.

Another friend took me to chemo cycle number four in the beginning of December. We parked ourselves in the corner of the ward and caught up. I went home and repeated the previous pattern of the three previous cycles: tablets, injections, emotions. I felt ill, I felt more ill, I felt depressed, I began to feel bored and then better.

Eleven days later I was on a train to see Calvin Harris in London with some friends. At knocking fifty I probably shouldn't have gone and eleven days post-chemo I definitely shouldn't have gone, but I did, an exquisite 'fuck you cancer' moment. I felt weak and fragile. I had no strength or spirit. My legs were slow and heavy. I sat down as much as possible. It was overwhelmingly busy and I felt confused with so many people and so much noise surrounding me. I felt overloaded; this was very different from my still and silent sofa days of the previous two months. From our balcony seats we could see the sea of people below us getting louder as the drink and music flowed, the atmosphere hypnotic as the DJs did their thing and lasers flashed around the venue. They all looked younger and healthier than me, lithe and energetic, full of life. It was good for my mind to get out and be reminded that the things I love and that make me who I am were still out there, but it was tough going, every breath required effort and every step strength, neither of which I had.

As much as my mind wanted to connect and experience the things that gave my life 'meaning' (page 322), my body wasn't ready and I felt I had put myself at risk by being determined to go.

CHAPTER 15

"What lies behind us, and what lies before us
are but tiny matters compared to what lies within us."

Ralph Waldo Emerson

My sadness seemed to peak around Christmas time, the second Christmas to be affected by cancer. That seemed unfair to me. I had done my time as a cancer patient, with cancer wrecking special days and times. I reminisced that this time last year we were in Australia. So much had changed and been lost since then. This time last year we were at the airport. This time last year it was hot and sunny. This time last year we were laughing with our family. This time last year we were at Manly Beach. This time last year we were in the Blue Mountains. This time last year we were at Noosa. This time last year I was happy. This time last year I didn't have cancer. This time last year I had hair. This time last year I wasn't shit scared.

Christmas somehow happened and I did the Christmas shopping bit by bit. Thankfully my nieces and nephews were happy with vouchers and cash. I made it easy for myself, shopping online and in supermarkets. I wasn't going to be able to provide the perfect Christmas, but it was the best I could manage under the circumstances. I was careful not to put myself at unnecessary risk with germs and bugs, and would wash my hands and use anti-bacteria gel at regular intervals. I was developing obsessive tendencies.

We were spending Christmas Day with Ian's family and enjoyed cards and gifts with childhood excitement amidst cocktails, crackers, tinsel and the twinkle of Christmas lights, in the darkness that is mid-winter and treatment for cancer. I took a moment to look around the room, three generations grateful to be together, no one was missing. We exchanged smiles, silently acknowledging this could have looked very different.

Another pocket of happiness which kept me going and reminded me of the good times I'd had. Ian had a book made up of photos from our trip to Australia as a Christmas present for me. I cried turning the pages, looking at blue skies, smiling faces and memories. I tried to focus on the thought that life could be like that again. We caught up with friends and family over the coming days. I found it stressful to focus and function at hosting and preparing food. I hadn't done much for the last few months and my brain felt frazzled and overloaded at the even tiniest decision. My abilities, confidence and concentration felt rocked. I felt and looked a tired mess.

The CT scan was repeated at the end of December and it showed the cancer had gone; departed, wiped out, killed off before it killed me. The chemo had done its job. This was important because, for the radiotherapy to have maximum effect, the tumour needed to have been as small as possible. I felt relieved and yet suspicious. How could something so large and dangerous seemingly vanish? Where was it? Was it lurking silently elsewhere? This was the medical evidence I needed and, coupled with my oncologist's words at the start of treatment, there was no reason why I couldn't have another ten years if I responded to treatment and, according to the CT scan, I had. In times of anxiety and uncertainty, I anchored myself back to these two pieces of information: the medical evidence and the words of someone who knew the facts; not my scared, crazy thoughts.

We spent New Year's Eve with friends walking round a lantern-lit Kew Gardens. We ate pizza and drank prosecco. It was informal, relaxed and I enjoyed it, my head covered with a knitted beret, concealing the other part of my life. I was looking forward to saying that I had had chemo last year in 2013 and that 2014 would hold something new for me. There was still the radiotherapy and recovery to go, but chemo was so very nearly last year.

I began to think about the year ahead and the plans we had made. We had booked to go and see Lovely Brother and his family in Sydney for February half-term in 2014. When the diagnosis came, I was not convinced the treatment would be finished by the departure date or, even if it had, whether I would be well enough to go. I began to make alternative plans to travel at Easter. A bonus would be we could go for longer, which meant we could add in a trip to New Zealand to visit friends who had left our village to return home there six months earlier. We researched changing the flights to Sydney, booking further flights to Auckland, as well as hiring a camper van, and explored a route that would take in as much of the North Island as is possible in a week. Happy days, a crazy 'fuck you' post-cancer treatment idea. It was very important for me to honour the arrangements I had made; it enabled me to feel that cancer hadn't got the better of me. Once we had the radiotherapy timetable, we would be able to make a firm plan. The idea of returning to Australia kept me going.

There were many moments of kindness from many people throughout the treatment, but the kindness and understanding of six friends stands out, genuine no bullshit friends whom I trusted with my life. Six people who don't know each other, but were my sturdy rocks when everywhere else in my life was quicksand. They were friends who during this time put my needs first and didn't ask anything in return of me, just that I survived. They genuinely wanted to be there in the way I needed. They put their needs and feelings on the back-burner to support me through mine. Sometimes they looked as scared as I felt, mirroring what I was feeling, but unable to say or show it. Each gave something different. Some of them have seen me go through cancer twice. They didn't abandon me. They didn't burden me. I had to find my own way through cancer and in my own time. They were people who I felt comfortable having a meltdown or sharing a crazy idea with, people who allowed me to be what I needed to be in that moment. I wasn't being judged or rescued or shut down. This was truly the greatest gift of all.

One gave me a charm necklace made up of my favourite things, which I wore to appointments. Another gave me a card made up of photos from the past twenty-five years of our friendship, which arrived on a day that I was feeling particularly low. It reminded me of the fun I'd had and the fun I would have again, and then I cried. I cried a lot, wanting to go back to or go forward to these fun times, to get out of the uncertainty and hideousness that I was currently living with and in. An avid reader and researcher regularly sent me cancer-related books, articles and links. Like her, they were honest and to the point, and not the fluffy bullshit stuff that is written about cancer. These offered realism and alternative, refreshing perspectives. She also had an acute sixth sense of when I was not okay, even though I proclaimed that I was. She just knew and would push me to tell all. I knew and she knew, so it made it easier to share when all was clearly not okay.

A friend who lives several hundred miles away would text every day and I knew I could call or visit at any time if I needed. Just knowing I could do this was comforting, a lifeline from hell. A local friend who is like a soft cuddly toy, the softest kindest person I know, would visit. She would cry and I would cry, I needed to cry at the shitness of it all and she cried with me, and then we would swear and quickly we would be giggling at the shitness of the shitness and our swearword combinations, which were mainly four letters and related to body parts. She came to visit soon after the second diagnosis, and we sat watching rain falling outside. I glanced up and there were hundreds of swallows circling the grey skies above. I had not seen them over the house all summer and now they congregated to leave and head south. Swooping and swishing, it was a sign of hope for me that life would return next year. I also knew I could pop round to my neighbour at any time.

I had met each of them at different places and times in my life. Each friend was part of my world and kept me tethered as I drifted solo in the world of cancer and waited until I returned, our bond deepened by the near miss. I never questioned our bond; I knew it was there, solid and safe. I could ask them anything. They were calm, kind and respectful. They adapted to my needs in my new world. We are still friends to this day. Our friendships are rock solid. They were there for me. I am there for them. Our friendship survived cancer.

Keeping connected to my 'social' (page 323) dimension was very important for my mental health when so much of my life was focused on being a cancer patient. These connections helped me from slipping into a deeper depression.

CHAPTER 16

"Each time we face our fear,
we gain strength, courage and confidence in the doing."
Theodore Roosevelt

How do you tell someone you have cancer? It is not easy to say you have cancer and it is not easy to hear. Cancer isn't a gentle word; it's a punch in the face. You just know that it's going to affect the person you tell. And you will see their reaction and in turn have to react to them.

During cancer number one I told everyone everything because I didn't have many boundaries in my life. I was open and honest and treated everyone the same, wanting everyone to know everything about me. These were lovely, but in some way naïve, qualities to have and ultimately left me vulnerable and exhausted. Our lives had quickly come to resemble an under-resourced call centre and our lounge an overflowing florist's shop. It was exhausting. Soon the volume of information became unmanageable because I felt I had to respond to each contact and manage their feelings without being aware of, or supported in, my own.

No matter what I told or to whom, no one was going to make this better or take away the situation, the thoughts and feelings around cancer, and ultimately my fear of my death. Only I was going to be able to manage and accept this myself. This was a tough lesson in life as we are used to asking for help, or someone may offer to help us; they may comfort us and try to take our pain away. Cancer isn't like that. Cancer is lonely and isolating, and ultimately no one can rescue us from death and our feelings about death; we have to make our own peace about these and, through therapy and living a meaningful life, I had partially done this.

Birth and 'death' (page 321) are two life events which we face on our own. We have no recollection about birth but an increasing awareness of death. We need to gain our own 'acceptance' (page 327) and 'meaning' (page 322) about death, but that process is not quick or easy.

Second time around I didn't want to support other people. Second time around I couldn't cope with the anticipation of that. Second time around I wanted to be sad and angry. Second time around I wanted to be free to do what I needed to do. Second time around there were many more people in our lives. Second time around a second strategy was devised, based on what I had learnt from the first time. It wasn't going to suit everyone, but it was going to suit me and as I was doing this shit, that's how it needed to be.

Close family and friends had the full story and regular updates. I trusted them to respect my wishes and support me. I divided other people into those who I thought were going to be of some help and support, and those who weren't. This was a generally swift and easy process, possibly ruthless. I sent an email to those who I thought would be of help or support, outlining the news and, if they wanted to, how they could help. Those who I thought would be less helpful, for whatever reason, as well as gossips and vultures, I let read about my diagnosis on Facebook with a request that I was not contacted. I relied on the village gossip networks to fill in the gaps. Some people respected this, some people were relieved by this and some people ignored this.

"Following recent tests I have a recurrence of cancer, treatment is starting soon. This is obviously a really stressful time and I would be grateful if people would not reply to this post and respect that at this time this is all the information I wish to disclose."

The post was short and to the point. I felt I was 'in control' (page 333), if not of the diagnosis and outcome, at least how I managed the flow of information.

Social media enabled me to provide open and clear communication whilst at the same time keeping myself at a safe distance. I didn't have to witness and then manage, respond to, rescue or support the shocked and crumpled faces before me. I couldn't take on the tears or the intrusive questions. I had my own role to be getting on with. Supporting other people would detract from my goals of shrinking the tumour and being there for Poppy and Bonnie. Anything that was going to detract from this needed to be parked or deleted.

It was much less draining to be able to choose and then manage what I said, when and to whom. It also put paid to gossip because everyone was delivered the same unambiguous facts at the same time, and therefore any change of these words written in black on a white screen was down to personal interpretation. I could respond when I wanted to, protecting myself, and giving as much or as little information as I needed to or wanted to.

I took some time to process each piece of information about my treatment so that I had worked out the impact it had on me and my feelings before I shared it. This enabled me to deal with the impact it had on others, because I had worked through my feelings and reactions before I announced any updates. Because I had processed my thoughts and feelings, I was more detached and less affected when others expressed their thoughts and feelings.

When the second diagnosis came through, one of my main concerns and focus of anger was not being able to work while having my treatment. My initial reaction was that I didn't want to stop working with the clients I had. I felt as if I was abandoning them and I was hoping they wouldn't abandon me because work was such a part of my purpose. I had waited a long time to find a job which I loved. The next thought was how I would tell my clients I had cancer, followed by how I would manage working while having the treatment, and still look after myself while being a good counsellor.

The humanistic model of counselling which I practise is based on an open and honest relationship and communication, so not disclosing what was about to happen to me felt uncomfortable and disrespectful to my clients. It was probably going to be very obvious very soon what was happening to me. However, working out how much to say so that the therapeutic relationship was not damaged, or clients felt they would have to care for me, was going to be potentially challenging. This news was going to change the relationship with my clients and I needed to be prepared for that.

I contacted my supervisor straight away to discuss. She was calm, kind and supportive and questioned me in such a way that I gleaned my own answers for the way forward by exploring the options and what felt comfortable for me. As the relationship with my clients is a professional one, disclosure would need to be handled differently to family, friends and village gossips. It was important when I disclosed my diagnosis and treatment that I was in a stable place to be able to respond to my client's reactions without breaking down. I would also need to allow time and space for them to explore the impact it may have on them and their sessions, as well as for discussing how it was for them to hear about my diagnosis and what they wanted and needed. My supervisor suggested that I include that this was a recurrence of cancer, which would hopefully create safety and stability for my clients in them knowing I had been through this before.

I had little time to process the maelstrom before I met with my clients again for their weekly sessions. My fear was that I was going to break down and cry in front of them. I found the words and spoke them in a practical and detached way, saying clearly and, I hope, calmly and without a wobble in my voice that I had a recurrence of cancer and I would be having some treatment over the next few months. I then explored their options with them to empower them to recognise they now had a choice. They could end their sessions with me, I could help them find another counsellor to work with, or we could carry on, but I would only be able to work two out of three weeks and that my appearance was going to be changing. I knew there would be a reaction from each of them to this news, but I had no idea what it would be. I braced myself. We explored how it had been for them to hear this news and each client chose to carry on with their sessions.

My clients will never know how much I appreciated being able to continue to work. It gave me a sense of reality and maintained my sense of purpose. Work proved to be a welcome distraction and it grounded me in the bigger picture of my life amidst the chaos. For a few hours a week I could focus outside of the whirring in my head and burden in my body, connection that meant I didn't entirely detach from who I was away from my cancer life. It was a fragile but important connection to my life where being a cancer patient wasn't my primary role. I could be Rebecca the counsellor. It reminded me of a life outside of cancer, the life I hoped I could return to.

I did not know how this chemo combo would affect me, or if I would be well enough to work but I hoped, and at times was desperate in my hope, that I would be able to. I soon learnt the rhythm of chemo cycles and my physical reactions to them. I would stockpile my energy for work days, resting before and after.

Clients would ask me how I was. I kept to the same format. I thanked them for asking after me and gave a short, factual response, ensuring that the focus of the session returned to them as soon as possible to maintain the boundaries of the counselling relationship.

I was very grateful to be able to carry on with the 'configuration of self' (page 332) as a counsellor away from the 'configuration of self' (page 332) as a cancer patient. This gave 'meaning' (page 322) and hope to my life.

From 3rd September 2005 up to and including 19th September 2013, the school run had been a nice way to punctuate the day with a little laughter, a bit of gossip and a chance to catch up with friends twice a day; smiles, banter, play dates and the Friday cake sale rota. The playground took on a whole new meaning once the news of my cancer diagnosis broke, filtering round the playground as cancer was filtering around me. I feared being different, glanced at, stared at, talked about, questioned, pitied or rescued. I developed the head-down-keep-moving strategy to avoid this, ducking, diving and weaving. Twice a day I felt vulnerable, as if I was going to be pounced on and forced into answering questions I didn't want to. There was avoidance, averted eyes and turned bodies as I passed, the awkward conversations about the weather when I clearly looked shit. Actually I didn't give a fuck about the weather. I just wanted this to be over, to know I was going to be okay.

There were also platitudes, the heroic sentences about my strength and ability to beat cancer. Literally, fuck off.

The playground became an exposing place of difference: different lives, different days, different looks, different worries and different choices. I didn't want to be publically ill, to die a public death, my demise being macabrely observed and documented, hushed tones and sympathetic looks. I didn't want to look an epic failure twice a day. I felt like a mouldy orange rotting in the fruit bowl of health and happiness surrounding me. I did a lot of bargaining and hoping. If it could just be okay until Bonnie left primary school, please, I could then just slide away quietly. How I craved those boring and mundane days, where my biggest worry was the availability of organic ham at the supermarket. I wanted to protect the girls and for everything to be normal. They didn't deserve this. I was apoplectic when someone asked Poppy where the cancer was, because I hadn't disclosed that information. Why you would put your desire to know where a cancer tumour was above the care of a twelve-year-old child, I will never know.

I hated feeling I was being seen as a 'victim' (page 328) and pitied, or that I had failed in working hard enough to keep cancer away, but some people triggered these feelings with their words and behaviour.

The girls and their needs were different the second time around. First time around I had got away without saying much about what was going on, because they didn't have the knowledge or understanding of what was happening. I could protect them with normality, silence, routine, outings to the park, ice cream, bedtime stories, cuddles and kisses. I said nothing of my hell. I had got away without questions about my appearance. They didn't notice and therefore didn't care about the amount or texture or style of my hair. There was no impact on them whether I had hair or not. Looks and hair were superfluous to their requirements.

I trusted they would ask when they wanted to know something. Poppy was three when she asked why I had one boob bigger than the other. She had noticed my left and my right were different. I gave a casual, factual and brief explanation, just the headline. I hid the fear and anxiety behind the headline. I let them look and touch and ask the questions. I have found children ask as much as they want to know until they understand, and then they stop. I also bought a book called 'Mummy's Lump' which soon became a favourite bedtime story. The soft words and accompanying illustrations take the reader through the treatments and side effects of breast cancer. It's simply told and leaves room for questions to be asked or not.

Fast-forward ten years and looks (both theirs and mine) were much higher up the agenda, as was their awareness and feelings. They were more aware and conscious of how I looked. Was I going to lose my hair? Was I going to be stared at? If I was being stared at, that would embarrass them. The wrong jeans, top or trainers – that was bad enough, but hair loss? It was excruciating for them and in turn painful for me to watch. I had failed them again. I felt rejected. To me I was still their mum. I would have loved them with no hair. I was going to be a cancer patient. I was going to have chemo. I was going to lose my hair. I was going to be an *embarrassment* to them.

My hair loss was something the girls found hard. It created difference. Difference creates discomfort and embarrassment. Difference potentially creates a social threat to a teenager. Rejection. Isolation. They were sensitive to the fact that I looked different, different to how I had looked, different to how the community and society we live in looks. They were concerned about how this would impact on them, whether they would be teased or questioned. I frequently heard through the winter of 2013 an anxious 'Mummy, can you put a hat on?' as we hovered near the door before going out, to cover up the source of difference and embarrassment. This hurt like a knife through my heart. I felt I wasn't good enough, that I was failing and I couldn't be what they needed or wanted.

I felt I was failing as my 'configuration of self' (page 332) of being a perfect mother because I was going to embarrass them with my changing looks and difference.

CHAPTER 17

"Strength does not come from physical capacity.
It comes from an indomitable will."

Mohandas Karamchand Gandhi

There were both emotional and psychological similarities and differences with cancers one and two. Powerful feelings of anger masked my other feelings during cancer first time around, protecting me from my sadness, fear, guilt and anxiety. Time, therapy and creating a meaningful life resolved these to some extent. Second time around, intense feelings of sadness, anxiety and fear arrived from the moment I found the lump. I went from carefree and happy to terrified within a moment, without the anger there to distract or disguise it. Nothing would or could soothe this fear and anxiety about what lay ahead. At times my feelings became all-consuming.

Recognising and processing my feelings second time around was undoubtedly easier because I had spent six years in therapy, so I knew the good, the bad and the ugly in my life and about myself. I was calmer and more focused, and had worked hard in therapy to explore what my anger was about and create a meaningful life. I looked after myself in better ways because I knew what I needed, what gave me purpose and meaning, and it was quite simple: I loved work, running a home, family, socialising and exercise. This was what I needed. If I had access to these, I was okay, happy, calm and satisfied. There were other things I liked, but these were the basics of my life, the foundations, the safe base to explore from and return to.

The therapy and training between cancers one and two gave me much more awareness of my feelings and needs, and I was not frightened of allowing, experiencing and expressing them. I trusted the process; they were necessary and they would pass, each was there for a reason. By doing this I would experience less emotional and psychological distress along the way than by trying to avoid or deny these feelings. Expressing them would get me to 'acceptance' (page 327) as soon as possible and back to the life I loved. I bypassed 'denial' (page 326); this was happening no matter what.

The second time around I knew what would be good for me and what not so. I knew what worked and what didn't. I knew what I would need and what I wouldn't. I knew what would help and what wouldn't. I knew I was going to feel tired and ill. I knew my lovely life was going to change and that a Friday night get together with friends or a 5k run at dawn was going to be missing from my life for a while. I knew that I was going to feel sad and angry, and hopeless and depressed. But I also knew that I would get through what lay ahead in the coming months. I would find a way. I also knew that I had a great support network. I knew I would need both time and space to withdraw and be alone and time to have human contact. I knew I might need help in the way of childcare. I knew I may have to ask for help. I knew that as much as I didn't want to, I was going to be vulnerable and fragile. I knew the bucket list would be on hold. I knew there was a risk of dying during the treatment. I knew I needed to look after myself. I knew I couldn't be all things to all people. I knew that some days I would just survive.

The second time around I realised how much I used bargaining to gain acceptance about what was happening, instead of spending hours and days distressed about what was out of my control. The second time around I wasn't pregnant. Both girls were at school so, by comparison, this was going to be a doddle and in some ways it was. It was autumn after all, so less daylight and warmth luring me outside. A plethora of reality TV shows were coming up. What could be more fun than lying around for days on end watching them, avoiding the dull grey landscapes outside? But it wasn't fun. Watching reality TV was hardly a meaningful purpose for my body and mind, which craved stimulation and engagement, activity and life. Choosing to sit and watch rubbish TV is a luxury to switch off addled, overloaded, tired bodies and brains. Lying on a sofa because you feel too ill to attempt anything else, for me, was mind-numbingly boring. I was capable and wanted to do more, but my body and my brain were both telling me this was the way forward; to rest, to relinquish, to just lay down, to heal. It felt like failing, giving up, not even trying. But I listened to my mind and my body, bargaining of course that it wouldn't be long until I was going out again on a Friday night and running along country lanes at dawn. Just get the treatment and recovery done as quickly and easily as possible. The busy, creative, achieving part of me was just going to have to lie down, give in and let the treatment and my body do its thing.

> *It was very depressing to do nothing. I suffered the 'loss' (page 325) of giving up parts of my life which gave me 'meaning' (page 322) to have the treatment and this affected the 'social' (page 323), 'personal' (page 324) and 'spiritual' (page 324) dimensions of my life.*

The second time around I was aware how intensely protective I felt over Poppy. She had only started secondary school a few days before the diagnosis. She was known and would have been well supported at primary school, which felt comforting, but she wasn't at primary school. She was at a big, new secondary school where I knew no one and most of the communication is conducted via email. I didn't know anyone who could check that she was okay. This was very different to the first time when these fierce feelings of mother lion protection were focused on Bonnie. I felt sad knowing I could not protect my children from what lay ahead over the coming weeks and months. I felt torn in wanting to protect the girls, but knowing I couldn't. I didn't want them to see me ill and weak, and I felt embarrassed for failing them with this second diagnosis.

My 'configuration of self' (page 332) of protective mum and my 'be perfect' driver (page 329) were really challenged during this time, which created anxiety and guilt.

Both times I was scared of dying, but I was more terrified with the second diagnosis because the location of the tumour meant the likelihood of metastatic and unsurvivable cancer was much higher, a step closer to the exit door of life, goodbye and thank you for having me. Potentially this was very serious, my long-term survival more precarious. I was less naïve and avoiding with cancer number two, and more informed thanks to Google and my time in various volunteering roles. I still didn't want to say goodbye to Poppy and Bonnie, and this was the source of my greatest fear and sadness. It was so intense and unbearable to think about, I was paralysed at times and unable to really live life. I felt I would have failed at motherhood if I didn't see them become independent adults.

The brutal statistics of my second diagnosis helped me focus on what was important and where to concentrate my time and energy.

There was a much greater sense of calm and acceptance, and less panic, second time around. I knew what I was in for. I trusted my oncologist and myself. I knew it was going to be tough, but I also knew I could do the treatment and recovery. I was familiar with the treatment, hospitals, care and routine, and the hours which would be spent waiting. I applied my previous knowledge and experience of cancer to this second diagnosis, which lessened the trauma and anxiety. I knew I had the skills to survive. Because I had trust in my oncologist and myself already in place, I was able to spend less time struggling with how I would physically manage the coming months, and could allow and experience my feelings, which enabled me to process them and gain acceptance. The diagnosis and treatment were happening and there was nothing I could do about it apart from have the treatment, hope for the best and be the best mum I could each day.

By having a trusting medical relationship with my oncologist already in place, I didn't have to establish this. I trusted him totally with my medical care which was freeing, emotionally and psychologically, and helped me move to 'acceptance' (page 327) of the diagnosis much quicker than the first time.

I knew second time around that I had had all the treatment available to me and asked fewer questions. I accepted more quickly and easily. The treatment path seemed clearer with fewer options available. Options lead to choices. Choices lead to consequences. Consequences lead to anxiety. Anxiety leads to 3am wonderings of whether the right choice has been made and the possibility of other options, choices and consequences; a vicious and unproductive cycle.

I wasn't worried that there may have been a better treatment out there to increase my life and therefore avoid 'death' (page 321).

Hope was very important for me while I was having my cancer treatment. It wasn't something I particularly cultivated, it was just there. However awful my current situation and however powerless I felt to change it, I always had hope that there would be better times ahead.

The focus of my hope shifted over time. Hope that the cancer wasn't really cancer. Hope that the cancer wasn't aggressive. Hope that the cancer hadn't spread. Hope that I would have a chance of treatment. Hope that the treatment would work. Hope that I would have more time with my children. Hope that the cancer wouldn't come back. Hope for a future. Hope for another bucket list and 'fuck you cancer' moments. My hope kept me focused and determined, especially when things were difficult. For the majority of the time I had hope for something future-orientated, but when things were so awful and there was little or no hope, life became unbearably sad and depressing. Thinking and planning for a future helped me have hope. I found it easier to plan ahead the second time around, and was determined I was going to have a future; the first time, I wasn't so sure. This second time around it just felt that everything was going to be on hold for a while.

One day the focus of my hope will need to change. One day there will be no clear scans or mammograms or treatment options, and my hope will change from having more health to not being in pain and having the opportunity to be able to say goodbye.

My hope helped me avoid how awful things really were and formed part of the 'denial' (page 326) and 'bargaining' (page 326). My hope also drove me forward, along with my 'self-actualisation' (page 331), that things would get better.

There was minimal anger second time around, and what there was I directed at potentially not being able to work and the interruption to my life meaning. I vented this in supervision, personal therapy and with friends and family. There was nothing I could do to change this. I was either going to be able to work or I wasn't. Clients would either come or they wouldn't.

The pay-off for less anger was that there was much more sadness second time around. Sadness at not being able to do the things that I loved and which gave my life meaning, the things that I had worked hard to find, things I appreciated and valued. Sadness at possibly having to say goodbye to those I love. Second time around I didn't want to avoid my sadness. I didn't want to fill my day being relentlessly busy or constantly angry. I didn't want to be rescued from my sadness. I wanted to experience and express it, because I knew this was the way to move on and live once again.

My sadness at what I was experiencing and fear for the future did overwhelm me at times, and I was detached and depressed. Standing back and observing sadness is hard for people to watch because they want to do something, anything. Anything so they don't have to witness the tears and maybe feel helpless in trying to stem or solve them. There is something uncomfortable and almost unbearable for people to see someone crying. There are some things in life, such as grief, that can't just be taken away or made better. The experiencing and expressing of the sadness is part of the process of reaching acceptance of our situation, and not expressing the sadness can lead to other issues as we work harder and harder to avoid these feelings. The greatest gift anyone ever gave me was the time and space to cry and not feel that I had to stop because it was uncomfortable for them to watch or be with. No emotion lasts forever; at some point we stop crying, just as we stop laughing. We don't laugh about a joke or funny story forever, just as we don't cry forever.

> *There was much more sadness the second time around because I wasn't focusing on the anger and the whirlwind of energy it created that I used to focus on; anything other than facing my thoughts and feelings. My sadness now focused around the possibility of having to say goodbye and not being able to do the things which gave my life 'meaning' (page 322).*

Who doesn't like a good laugh, whether with friends, watching a comedy or at an ironic situation? Humour is a big part of my life. I love nothing more than a good giggle and belly laugh. However, there is absolutely nothing funny about cancer or having cancer. So therein lies a problem, how do we balance humour within the seriousness of a situation? It is socially unacceptable to joke about cancer and its side effects. Humour in the wrong context or setting can be degrading, insensitive and inappropriate, as well as hurtful. However, humour can allow us to talk about embarrassing, frightening, sensitive or difficult experiences. This can reduce their emotional and psychological impact, as well as isolation and tension, and increase connection, empowerment and how we manage adversity. The setting and context of the use of humour needs to be taken into account. Anecdotes, jokes, or during a conversation? Between friends, medics, doctors and patients, or between patients? Who initiates the jokes? Does humour require equality?

Humour was part of my life before cancer, so I needed to find a place for it during and after cancer. I laughed many times at just how awful cancer was. Following treatment I met a lady I hadn't seen for a while. She commented on my short haircut and I remarked that it was caused by chemo and was not through choice. I was laughing when I said it. She wasn't sure how to respond and was possibly embarrassed. Freud discusses laughter as a defence, as a middle-ground, a halfway house between recognising the seriousness of a situation and not being able to explore it or engage with it. It felt important that I made the jokes and not that I was joked at, about or with. Other people initiating jokes riled me, but then, looking at my part, I possibly invited their cancer joking as I joked about my experiences of cancer. Maybe it was better to say nothing, to be sombre and scared, but then that isn't really me.

We all experience anxiety at times. After having cancer the first time, I spent many hours and many days feeling anxious about the cancer returning, endless 'what ifs?' What if this? What if that? What if this and that? The anxiety only lessened as my confidence grew, time passed, life was lived and the cancer didn't return. But then I began to think of this differently. The anxiety shifted focus. The more time that passed, surely the risk of recurrence was more likely? Second time around I made a conscious effort not to worry early on, as the scans and blood tests had shown that I had had a total response to the treatment, so logically I had nothing to worry about.

> *I was able to balance my anxiety with 'logical' (page 332) and medical facts, and this enabled me to enjoy my life and focus on things I could 'influence and control' (page 333).*

The second time around, I found it much easier to accept help and support when it was offered, as well as say no when it wasn't what I needed. My loathing of being seen as a victim and asking or accepting help was extremely difficult. I felt a failure needing help, weak by asking, uncomfortable accepting and vulnerable that it may be taken away from me if I did accept it. However, in all that I had learnt in therapy, I began to recognise that people wanted to help me just as I enjoyed helping other people. It was a nice feeling to accept their help instead of feeling a failure by doing so. I began to trust people. I began to take a risk and ask for something small on a practical level, such as bringing the girls home after school. When this felt okay, I began to take bigger risks with my emotions, such as to say when I was sad or scared. To my delight, people were there and it felt good knowing that.

> *Following experiencing a 'secure attachment' (page 316) in therapy, I was able to understand what a safe*

*relationship felt like and be able to take emotional
risks within this. Gradually my 'be perfect' (page
329) and 'be strong' drivers (page 329) functioned
less, and a more vulnerable 'configuration of self'
(page 332) emerged.*

We all look for reasons, patterns and correlations to
explain things and create understanding and acceptance,
and a diagnosis of cancer is no different. Why did I get
cancer? Why didn't I get Parkinson's or have a stroke? Why
haven't my friends had cancer? Why did I get breast cancer
and not pancreatic cancer? Why did I get cancer in my
thirties and forties, and not in my twenties or seventies?
Was I just unlucky? Did I increase my risks with previous
lifestyle choices? Do I have dodgy DNA or was it because
I was meant to write this book? I don't know and nor does
anyone else. We know if we put our hand in the flame it
will burn and hurt, so we don't do it. We know if we can't
ski we don't begin with a red run. We take avoiding action
not to get hurt. Avoiding cancer is an area which doesn't
fit with our previous knowledge and understanding of
the world, and this can leave us feeling anxious, helpless,
powerless and out of control. If we don't know why we got
cancer, how can we avoid it again? Because these feelings
create distress, we seek to stabilise ourselves and can spend
time and money searching for why we got cancer and what
we can do not to get it again.

The first time around I didn't really look at why I had
got cancer. I focused on what I thought I could do not to
get it again. I didn't want any regrets: if only I hadn't eaten
this or drunk that. I actively and purposefully led a healthy

life full of fruit, veg, vitamins, fresh air and exercise. I didn't drink alcohol and I was happy with my choices as I felt I was doing what I could do to reduce the risk of a recurrence. That was until I reached the golden five-year post-diagnosis anniversary, the milestone, the anniversary that cancer campaigns proclaim that if cancer hasn't claimed you by then, you are free, safe, dismissed, discharged. I had done my time. I grew complacent and began to binge drink every so often, but maintained a healthy diet and weight, and exercised regularly. I felt safe. I could take a risk. I felt less controlled by the fear. I wanted to feel out of control. The trigger was music. If there was dancing involved I'd be drinking. I could go months without drinking, but then would drink to feel reckless, unpredictable and out of control. And I loved it. I loved letting go. I loved the freedom from constraint. I loved feeling free from the fear of cancer.

> I had spent so long trying to 'control' (page 333) so much that was 'out of control' (page 333), it was exhausting. Going out drinking and dancing was a way to manage and counteract this. I had still not addressed my underlying feelings of sadness and 'anger' (page 326) at the 'loss' (page 325) and 'trauma' (page 332) I had experienced, so binge drinking was another way of trying to manage this.

Cancer the second time around was different. I wondered what I had done or not done for the cancer to return. Was it the binge drinking or the switch to soya yoghurt a few months earlier? Was it the grief and depression following our beloved and young dog dying? Was it the loss from my life of my lovely brother and a close friend moving abroad? Was it the stress from an extension we had built which resulted in a protracted court case, or the loss of purpose following the end of the counselling course? Or was it just that cancer had found a way to morph and grow again and work around the tamoxifen? Again, no one can answer those questions for me and the not known is hard to manage and accept, but to keep searching for the reasons creates anxiety and pressure. Each second I spend on searching, I am not living and enjoying. I counteract these feelings by living each and every second with purpose and passion.

The second time around I looked more deeply at the emotional aspects of my life and, although I had addressed much in my personal therapy and counsellor training, there was still more to do. I live with even less stress and anxiety now. I walk away from the dramas instead of starting them. I meditate and relax daily, resting both my body and my mind. I respect my mind and body more now and care for them equally. Some stress is okay and can be used positively, creating a surge of energy to achieve a task, but it also serves as a warning sign that something is not right. Relentless stress which we cannot resolve can be damaging to our health. I am in no way suggesting stress is linked to cancer, but it saps our energy, energy that can be spent in other ways, more productively.

I took responsibility for what I could change. My 'self-actualisation' (page 331) drove me to continually improve; to be as happy as I could be.

I am a massive fan of the NHS but, because of my anxiety of the unknown during both cancers, felt I wanted to take an active role and responsibility in my treatment. Being passive is not my style, particularly when my life is potentially at stake. I became an amateur expert in my illness, treatment, options and research. I couldn't control cancer, but what I could do was become informed so I could ask questions to create understanding, empowerment and equality in the medical relationships. I asked and researched enough to feel I understood, but not enough to feel out of control or scared. I attended every appointment with an awareness of the purpose of the appointment, the research around the topic and roughly what needed to happen. This gave me a sense of participation and I felt educated in my health. I wanted to show I cared and hopefully they would care that I cared, and in turn care. Through this involvement, I have grown in confidence and assertiveness.

As time has passed I have learnt to reassure myself, to talk and soothe myself, to meld both logic and emotion. I feel well and I have no symptoms. I take my medication and attend medical appointments. This is what I can control. This is what I can take responsibility for. Unless I start choosing lifestyle factors such as smoking and drinking, which will increase my cancer risk, this really is all I can do. I don't believe I have any control over if, where or when the cancer returns, but I can live my life fully between now and then.

Instead of feeling overwhelmed and trying to control everything, I looked at what I could take responsibility for and let go of what I had no 'control' (page 333) over.

CHAPTER 18

"Don't count the days. Make the days count."

Muhammad Ali

Following the fourth and final chemo cycle, I was placed on a maintenance treatment of goserelin and letrozole, which I would be staying on until it failed; that is until I had a recurrence, or I made it to ten years. My cancer had needed hormones to grow and so the aim of the treatment was to have the least number of hormones possible circulating in my body, to give the cancer less of a fuel supply. I would now be in a medically induced menopause. A menopause created this way is abrupt and intense, whereas during a natural menopause the level of hormones declines over a few years. The menopause occurs in females when their ovaries stop producing eggs because of a reduction in the levels and production of sex hormones. This can happen either naturally (at around the age of fifty) or because of medical treatment such as treatment for cancer. Most women experience physical and emotional changes during this time, such as hot flushes, tiredness, weight gain and depression. Some women may take HRT (hormone replacement therapy) to replace the declining hormones and alleviate the menopausal symptoms. HRT is not suitable for everyone and especially anyone with hormone dependent breast cancer.

The goserelin is implanted under the skin over my stomach once a month, having applied skin-numbing cream to the implant site an hour before. Apparently the needle via which it is implanted is pretty large. I've never looked and I have no intention of doing so. The nurses' faces and slight hand shake in the moments before the implant are enough to tell me. An alternative is to undergo an oophorectomy (the surgical removal of the ovaries) or they could be radiated out of action, but I wasn't keen for any more general anaesthetic or radiation to be coming my way unless it was absolutely necessary and there was no other alternative.

Letrozole is a tablet, taken daily, and is an aromatase inhibitor used to treat hormone receptive breast cancer in menopausal women who have either been through the menopause naturally, surgically or medically (see goserelin above). In post-menopausal women, the main source of oestrogen is through the conversion of androgens (sex hormones produced by the adrenal glands) into oestrogens. This process is carried out by an enzyme called aromatase and happens mainly in the fatty tissues of the body. Letrozole (as well as other aromatase inhibitor medicines) block this process and the cancer cells dividing.

This drug combo is physically difficult and I have really suffered with pain and stiffness in my joints, and for the first few months would literally seize up after a period of inactivity. Some nights I would have to crawl to bed after watching an hour or so of television. I tried several supplements to no avail and reluctantly accepted that this was how it was going to be. My oncologist recommended I kept moving, moving and more moving. I didn't want to pass comment that this was the bit that hurt and that I didn't want to move ever again, but he was, of course, right. This is the first time that I have made the menopausal journey, but he, of course, has seen it hundreds of times and in this medical way. I can now recognise the stiffness starting and a quick ankle twist or shoulder roll gets things moving again. As time has passed, so has the stiffness. There were other physical changes to my downstairs lady garden, but I will spare you the details; let's just say that with a further prescription from a gynaecologist, all is in good working order again.

I had always been slim and putting on a menopausal stone was difficult to accept, and counting calories was not something I was used to. Shifting it seemed impossible. I did some Googling and researched the calories I'd need as a nearly fifty-year-old menopausal woman. 1,300 per day. I then proceeded to Google what 1,300 calories looked like in food format. I was horrified, it was hardly anything. I'd easily get through 1,300 calories a day just in chocolate and latte. Some unpleasant changes were ahead, but in life we can get used to anything if we want the goal enough. So extra-super-healthy eating would be required, as well as regular exercise, not just throughout the week but throughout the day, which helped both my joints and my waistline. Every calorie consumed or used would count. Squats while I cleaned my teeth, walking and cycling where and when I could. I cut down on carbs and upped my raw veg intake.

The emotional aspects of the menopause were more difficult to manage and control; less obvious, less visual. Low mood became the depressing norm and was as difficult to shift as my expanding waistline. I spent a good year with thoughts of not wanting to go on, just drifting off to sleep and not having to face my lack of energy and focus anymore. I am now careful to plan my days and weeks to include what makes me happy: friends, exercise and fresh air, trips to explore and experience new destinations. I also set myself both short- and long-term goals to keep me focused and to keep the depression at bay.

It's not just the cancer that impacts one's life; the ongoing treatments take their toll, both physically and mentally. The changes can be difficult to accept, manage and live with.

The 'acceptance' (page 327) of change and the consequences that I didn't want, or hadn't chosen, was difficult. I was very depressed at this time and felt my life was 'meaningless' (page 322), as so much had been taken away while I was being treated and, although physically I was doing more, I hadn't recovered emotionally or psychologically.

I was referred for radiotherapy in early January 2014 and met Mr Radiologist, a nice man at hospital number two. I went prepped with a list of questions. First up was exploring why surgery was not an option, to create understanding and soothe my angst. He explained calmly and clearly that there were numerous important bits and bobs in the area of the supraclavicular fossa and it would be impossible to find the affected lymph node and remove it safely without the risk of damaging the surrounding important bits and bobs. I understood and therefore could accept this. We were off to a good start. I also wanted to know what would happen if I had a recurrence, because I was aware that, once you have had radiotherapy, a repeat dose to the previously treated area is not an option. He said that recurrence is very rare to an area which had been treated with radiotherapy. This coupled with the clear CT scan in December was the reassurance I needed, and I could move on as I understood the reasons behind the treatment choices.

Understanding what was happening to me and what my options were created both empowerment and safety. This enabled me to have 'acceptance' (page 327) about what was happening and not feel angry, sad, hopeless or helpless.

Mr Radiologist examined me and referred me back to hospital number three for radiotherapy treatment. Treatment had changed from the first time around and instead of twenty-five sessions of radiotherapy, fifteen were now given. Anxiety increasing. But the medical world being the medical world, there would have been research conducted to provide evidence for this reduction to happen. Anxiety decreasing. Life and plans became suspended, waiting for the radiotherapy planning session date to be arranged.

The format of the radiotherapy planning session had also changed and was now conducted by CT scan instead of X-ray. The staff hadn't changed though, and the lady running the planning session remembered me from ten years ago, when she was newly qualified. She was more excited about this than me; I just wanted to get on and get home, but that was not to be. Because of the timings of the radiotherapy appointments, and being at two different hospitals, my case notes had not been heard at this hospital's MDT meeting (multidisciplinary team meeting, where every cancer patient is discussed by a team of specialists to consider treatment options). And because my case had not been heard at the MDT meeting, no one had called for the notes to work out the positioning of this course of radiotherapy to ensure it would not overlap the site where the previous radiotherapy had been given. This meant that there was going to be a wait, probably a very long wait, while they tried to retrieve the notes which would have to be couriered over from a storage site. If they could not retrieve the notes, it would mean a return trip for the planning session. I began to cry.

We agreed I would return at 2pm to see if my notes had been successfully retrieved. This was stressful enough without further unexpected delays. I was fragile and vulnerable. Something as simple as a delay was enough to trigger my tears. I returned at 2pm and thankfully the notes had arrived. A weak, tearful smile crept across my face.

Writing how I had cried because my notes weren't present feels pathetic, but this speaks of how fragile I was feeling.

The appointment began with me stripping off and lying on a CT bed, just for a change. Several pairs of eyes were looking at me. I felt like I was a specimen in a giant petri dish. The treatment area was agreed and mapped out, and the dose was calculated, checked, approved and fed into a computer to be retrieved fifteen times, beginning the following week. I was bored with even the thought. Beam me up and fast-forward. But of course that can't be done, you have to live and experience the daily tedium of being a cancer patient on your own; it's not something you can pass on, contract out or opt out of.

I attended the first appointment a week later, where I was given the timetable for the fifteen sessions. I had to do a little reshuffling to fit in school pick-ups and work, but it was doable. The radiotherapy treatment centre had grown since the last time I was here and there were now six machines instead of four; six machines zapping six patients an hour, eight hours a day, five days a week. The session times were streamlined and maximised. You now got changed into your dressing gown in a cubicle outside of the treatment room before entering the room for treatment. However, I didn't own a dressing gown, which seemed to cause some gasps, shock and horror. I suggested that I was not about to purchase one, especially for this. After a discussion with other nurses, the nurse conceded that I could wear a vest top and roll it down to be treated.

And so the daily commute began; the driving, the parking, the walking, the waiting, the changing, the name checking, the positioning, the repositioning, the abandonment, the aloneness, the treatment, the beams, the whirring, the click, the end of the treatment, the getting dressed, the returning to the remainder of the day, the tiredness, the conserving of energy, the resting, the struggle, the boredom, the repetition, the monotony, the resentment, the tick of the list, a day and a treatment closer to resuming my life where my primary role and occupation wasn't being treated for cancer.

Family and friends had offered to take me to the radiotherapy. People wanted to help and that was kind and I was open to this. However, trying to coordinate treatment times, diaries and my own commitments became a stressful task and a logistical challenge. So I abandoned the idea and drove myself, meeting friends either before or after treatment to break the monotony.

Each of the fifteen treatments lasted for approximately thirty seconds, sandwiched centrally in a two-hour door-to-door round trip. This invisible treatment is different to other cancer treatments because it is visually barren; there are no tubes or needles, no trays of drugs, just nakedness under the beam of green light. As the treatments progressed, a perfect pink and then red square defined the area which was being treated, marking the site that had been so carefully calculated and coordinated. A replica was also forming on my shoulder, where the silent and invisible beams had passed through my skin, bones, flesh and blood, creating an exit site; so accurate, so perfect, created with mathematical precision.

The final treatment day arrived. I wore a pink coat as if to brighten the winter's day and celebrate my freedom. A friend came with me to the midday appointment and, after the final radiotherapy treatment, we went for a celebratory lunch with accompanying glass of fizz. I expected to feel happy, but I didn't. I felt detached and distant, robotic in my behaviour. It felt wrong to celebrate the end of something I didn't want to do in the first place.

I was relieved that the oncology timetable had ended and I was free once more, free to pick up the pieces of my life and carry on. Just where were the pieces of my life? What do you do the day after you finish treatment for cancer? How can you switch from cancer patient to… to what? I needed time to adjust, time to heal, time to recover, time not to be traumatised, time to feel safe, time to work out who I was now and was going to become, time to work out how cancer had affected me this time.

I slipped gently and quietly back into my life. There was no big party or celebration. I was exhausted. It was difficult to experience my constantly changing thoughts and feelings, searching for something but I didn't know what. I felt pointless. I had done the tough part, modelled the fighter, the survivor, the strong one who beat cancer. Again. There was a sudden rush of anxiety about all the jobs I had put off while I was having my treatment, and I diverted my attention and feelings to these, because looking at how cancer had affected me was too difficult. I got busy doing jobs. I had a purpose and felt I was achieving. I felt in control. But I was, of course, avoiding experiencing and processing the feelings and trauma which had just occurred.

I became very practical and gained a sense of achievement and purpose, as per 'stage 3' (page 318) and 'stage 4' (page 318) and to avoid stagnation as in 'stage 7' (page 319). Thinking about the emotional impact of the 'trauma' (page 332) would have been too much as this point.

Six weeks after the end of the treatment I was steadily recovering, but nowhere near fit. I could just about get through the day without being overcome with tiredness. My nails split very easily and I could walk and cycle for short periods of time, but was not able to run or lift weights, which I missed. My hair was short and thin and was taking longer to grow back than I remembered the first time, but I did have a full set of eyelashes. I checked hair growth progress daily, searching for signs of change and its return to its lush pre-chemo status. I photographed my head from several angles and compared images at forensic levels. I felt less attractive, sexy and confident than I did before but I also knew I wouldn't feel like this forever.

I used 'bargaining' (page 326) to gain 'acceptance' (page 327) that, although I couldn't undertake my beloved running, I could cycle and walk. This enabled me to avoid engaging with the 'anger' (page 326) which I might have experienced about this.

At the end of March, the radiotherapy team signed me off. This appointment was immediately followed by an appointment with the oncology team, just across the corridor. I can be as logical as I like but there is still an element of anxiety and unknown about these appointments. Both the clinical and medical oncology teams looked at me and declared health. I wondered what was happening at a smaller, less detectable level: the cells. What were my cells up to? Was the assassin hiding and recruiting other cells, waiting to grow again, sneaking up silently somewhere else?

No one could feel any lumps and bumps, which was a huge relief. I felt I could breathe and relax, at least for the time being. Two medical teams, separated by a corridor and a few minutes in time, had said the same. The next day I would not have two medical teams declaring my health, and I would have to reassure myself when the anxiety would sweep in like a sea fog, spreading doubt.

Unfortunately the treatment had taken its toll on my bones and, following a scan to check my bone density, I now had osteoporosis (a condition which weakens the bones making them fragile and more likely to break). I would be given an annual infusion of zoledronic acid to prevent further bone density loss, which also reduces the risk of secondary bone cancer (where breast cancer cells migrate from their original site and begin to grow on bones). My oncologist ran through the possible side effects and I consented to the treatment. It was lovely seeing him again. I felt proud at getting to the end of my treatment and I wanted to show him how well I'd done – the good patient who'd survived.

I left the hospital and deeply breathed in the fresh spring air, bright and blue. I caught wafts of fragrant spring scent. Somewhere in the background, a lawnmower was making the first cut of the year. I felt I had permission to live again. My body was safe and disease-free. It was hard to believe that just six weeks beforehand, I was having the radiotherapy treatment and twelve weeks beforehand my last chemo. The treatment was four months in total and seems such a short amount of time in comparison to the length of my life, but there were minutes that felt like hours, hours that felt like days and days that felt like years. I bargained that if four months out bought me even four years of life, it was worth it.

CHAPTER 19

"The real voyage of discovery consists
not in seeking new landscapes, but in having new eyes."

Marcel Proust

I was fed up with feeling stiff and 140 years old, overweight and without my lush thick hair. Maybe I should have appreciated my health and my hair more when I had them both. I felt frumpy and unattractive, with an underlying moodiness and depression. My focus had quickly shifted from gratitude for health and life, to frustration about minor inconveniences and my looks. I met again with the amazing image consultant for a well-timed spring/summer clothes shop. I was feeling increasingly negative about my body and my body shape, and hated every single item of clothing I possessed. Her objective perspective was that, yes, I had put on weight, but it was evenly spread and that I had gone from a size 8/10 to a 10/12, and that was okay;

I was knocking 50 after all! If I covered my face up and looked at my underwear-clad body I actually looked okay. There was no cellulite, there was just more of me and I needed to tweak what I bought. Two bags of clothes from Debenhams later I felt more confident and sparkly.

Knowing I looked good in what I wore built and maintained my self-confidence, which cancer had affected.

We set off for our trip to Sydney a few days later: the two long flights, hours of movies watched on mini-screen inches from our eyes, the soundtrack interrupted with announcements, zooming through time zones, day becoming night and then day again, trolleys of food and drink passing by, breakfast served at lunchtime and dinner for breakfast, followed by another breakfast, smiles and babies crying, counting down the hours and minutes to see my family, the sun and the stunning beaches, the fresh air and freedom, the freedom from being a recovering cancer patient, the long customs' queues holding us back, the moment of reunion when your eyes meet in arrivals, the hugs, the tears, the relief, the catch-ups which are as special as they can get, especially when cancer has threatened the possibility.

Lovely Brother collected us from the airport and we drove to their house on the spectacular Sydney coastline. We stopped in the early morning sunshine at Maroubra Beach, watching the waves arriving on the beach in the warm and windless air. The UK and cancer already seemed a million miles away. We had a lovely few days in Sydney.

There were cousin catch-ups, giggles and escapades with rotas for bunkbed positions, sightseeing, delicious dining and relaxing.

We left a few days later to begin the New Zealand leg of our trip, arriving in Auckland and collecting the camper van to begin our winding journey south to Masterton. I'm great at big crazy ideas and Ian is brilliant at planning at a more detailed level, and has much more patience than me at researching, comparing and booking resorts and accommodation. He created an itinerary of spectacular views, stunning sunsets, open roads and deserted campsites. We would travel in the early part of the day to our next destination, in time for lunch followed by an afternoon of sightseeing and arriving at our next night's accommodation, in time to set up before dark. Wherever we went, so did the camper van and it led to some interesting supermarket car park manoeuvres and plenty of good laughs. The vastness and magnificence of the country really struck me. The tranquillity and beauty of Lake Taupo and the strength of the ocean and remoteness at Cape Palliser will stay with me forever. My anxiety and mind settled with the beauty and calmness around me.

We returned to the UK towards the end of April, and a few days later I was scheduled for a day out at hospital number one for a mammogram, goserelin implant and the first zoledronic acid infusion. I felt I had taken a step back. I began to realise that once a cancer patient, always a cancer patient. I was never far from a cancer treatment, test, appointment or cancer-related thought.

The mammogram and goserelin implant passed

without incident. Next up was the zoledronic acid infusion. I had saved the best till last. I had not had the zoledronic acid before and it was set up to be administered as for chemo. Name check and match with drug tray contents, vein found, skin cleaned, cannula inserted, saline flushed, drug bag hung, pump set, arm out, held straight and still on a freshly-laundered, crisp, white pillow. I felt sick as my mind connected with the previous chemo experiences and I could feel the cold fluid enter my vein one drop at a time until the bag had emptied and the pump proclaimed this by beeping. Then another saline flush, after which the cannula was removed and the hole in my hand covered by a cotton wool ball and then plastered over, advertising that a medical procedure had just taken place.

I had been advised about the possible side effects as part of the consent procedure. I usually don't pay attention to descriptions of side effects because the thing with side effects is, usually, they are very personal; you are never quite sure if you are going to experience them or not and, if so, to what level. After twenty-three hours I had the side effects just as they had been outlined. I felt shocking, and every bone in my body ached. My face was red like a tomato. I was hot and then cold, and then hot and then cold, and then hot and then cold, and then the hot again. I turned to Google for reassurance – potentially I was going to feel like this for two weeks. Thankfully I didn't and I felt better the next day.

During my treatment I had stumbled upon a mindfulness retreat in a counselling magazine. The course was running 15th–19th May. My brain was desperately searching and craving for a way to switch off, to stop the constant whirring. I was searching for seemingly elusive stillness, calm and quiet. The timing of the course seemed perfect and, similarly to the Bristol Cancer Centre Course, would form a self-care ending to the treatment of cancer, which would end on my last day of being forty-eight years old; it felt timely. Unfortunately, despite enquiring seven months' before the course would run, it was already fully booked. Not wanting to give up hope, I asked to go on the waiting list. I had an inner sense of knowing that I would be going. It was meant to be and two weeks before the course start date, a place became available.

After lots of planning, list making and organising, I set off to Dorset in the glorious late spring sunshine with the trees and birds bursting into life all around me. I arrived at the retreat a few hours later. The countryside setting, the simply furnished rooms, the indoor pool and the symbols announcing the activities all added to the experience, detoxing our minds, from what distracted us and consumed us. It was nurturing and nourishing.

The course leaders encouraged us to leave our lives and coping strategies behind. We were invited not to: leave the site (epic fail, I couldn't resist the lure of the gorgeous countryside which surrounded the retreat); consume alcohol (pass); use technology (major fail); read (minor fail); watch TV (pass); or talk (pass). I totally LOVED every second I spent in silence, although it meant something different to us all; for some the silence felt punishing. I discovered silence was what I needed and what had been missing from my life, the off button for my hyperactive and hyper-vigilant brain. And yet I was still surrounded by and connected to people, it was not lonely or isolating.

I liked being near people but not having to make the effort of conversation. I was excused from making and engaging with small talk, which I find tiring and, at times, boring.

Over the next few days, by de-junking the noise that I was constantly bombarded with, I learnt to listen to my body. Other senses had a chance to be heard. I began connecting with my other senses that had been drowned out for years by my constant thinking. Our days were filled with mindful activities and I became increasingly aware of sensations and feelings in my body. The more I switched off the noise in my head and tuned my focus to my body, the more I began to notice the aches, the anxiety, the birdsong, the sights, colours, sounds and smells that were all around me, which I was permanently speeding past to avoid having to stop and feel. It was a delight to notice and feel, from noticing nothing to noticing everything. My favourite activity was the barefoot walking meditations around the retreat; stopping regularly to notice what my five senses were telling me. Feeling connected to the earth beneath me was wonderful, as well as grounding, and to this day I still walk mindfully and slowly round the garden, stopping and noticing, escaping for a few moments from my busy mind.

The vegetarian food was exquisite and in every sumptuous mouthful you could taste the love and passion it had been prepared with. I didn't want to swallow it because I enjoyed tasting it so much.

We took turns with the chores. Each was pleasurable because we weren't being distracted by noise; we were feeling what we were doing. I walked in the surrounding countryside, past flint-built barns and flower-draped walls and through shady narrow lanes. Suddenly I felt alive again, alive as the land I was walking on. Four glorious days of sunshine filled with awareness, self-love and self-care, savouring moment by moment. It felt symbolic that the course ended during an enormous thunderstorm and torrential rain, an ending and a beginning.

I reluctantly packed up my things and got in my car with tears in my eyes, sad to leave this tranquil and restorative place. I wanted to leave the anxious and angry Rebecca behind; it was refreshing to realise, after forty-eight years, that I could, that I had a choice. I left the retreat more in tune with myself, sensitive and softened, detoxed from my anxiety and anger. I didn't want to go back to the person I had arrived as. I drove along the narrow country lanes towards the main road and felt I had returned to another world. The busyness of the roads and the constant processing of information and making decisions overwhelmed me during the drive home. People's faces looked so strained and tense, as if they were going to erupt like volcanoes at any point. These faces were a reminder of who I didn't want to be anymore. I didn't want to rush anywhere ever again. I had missed so much by doing so, so many beautiful, simple things; feeling the ground as I walked, chewing, feeling and tasting food which I would previously gulp down without experiencing. Sometimes I didn't even remember eating, as I was rushing to the next activity, to achieve the next goal.

I cried on and off for the next twenty-four hours as I began to recognise what was wrong with my life. I used being busy to avoid and distract myself from feeling vulnerable and frightened. I had been addicted to sex, drama, excitement, flirting, food, fags, texting, rubbish relationships, friends and social media, but now I was becoming addicted to the feelings of calm and peace. If I was going to create these, I was going to have to change. Any change requires letting go of something. I used to use the dramas to feel alive and attract attention, but I could now feel alive from taking a breath or watching the beauty of the world around me, reading a couple of pages, feeling the long grass brush on my legs or hearing dry, crunchy soil under my feet, drinking a mug of steaming latte or watching waves on a beach, each simple and yet rich. By knowing what felt good I could change what didn't.

The mindfulness course is where I really began to address my 'anger' (page 326) and anxiety, not just from what cancer had created but from other events and areas in my life. I didn't want to feel like that anymore and the retreat had detoxed me from these feelings. I changed significantly at this point and, in turn, so did my relationships. Many of them were built on excitement and fun, but ultimately fear and anxiety, but I wanted relationships built on love, safety and security, as per 'stage 6' (page 319).

Mindfulness added richness and harmony to my life and it complemented the work my counsellor had done with me. I no longer wanted to rescue people, making myself indispensable to them. I now knew what my values, likes and needs were. I was now able to walk away if these weren't met or respected. I no longer lived seeking the next adrenalin fix wherever I went, with no awareness of the consequences, hurt or path of destruction which I left in my wake. Yes I was fun, yes I was lively, yes I was exciting, but in the long term this was not such a fun way to live. The feelings I gained from the dramas were temporary. I now had something unpredictable living in my life with me over which I had no control and which wasn't going to go away. I didn't need to be adding in more drama and chaos. I needed to change in order to steady up and stabilise the imbalance of cancer. I couldn't then, and can't now, get rid of cancer, but I can choose the amount of drama and chaos I add in. I like the analogy that we all live with seven dustbins and only six lids: we are permanently living with something uncomfortable; once we deal with an issue, another quickly takes its place. Cancer is my bin without a lid. I didn't want any more bins without lids, anything else unpredictable in my life, and that included me.

Here I began to work out what I could take responsibility for and recognise the consequences of my choices.

I awoke the next day as a forty-nine year old. For some reason I was reluctant to celebrate my birthday. Previously I had always been big on celebrating and acknowledging I had lived for another year, proclaiming life and that cancer hadn't claimed me. The day quietly passed. I now craved peace and quiet, calm and solitude. I now knew I could not go back to the drama and anger.

CHAPTER 20

"One day you will hear the sound of time rustling
as it slips through your fingers like sand."

Sergei Lukyanenko

Four months after my treatment had finished I felt physically okay most of the time. At the time I didn't think I would recover from my lethargic days spent on the sofa, watching TV and eating sausage rolls. I am now more careful how I spend my energy and plan the day. If I'm going out in the evening, I take a rest in the afternoon. Previously I would have viewed this as an immense failure that I had not achieved all 400 things on my to-do list by 6am, but now it's okay. I look after myself more, my priorities have changed. Part of me still feels tethered in the world of cancer, unable to free myself and escape. There are days during which I don't think about cancer as much and there are days when I think of nothing else, repeatedly checking my body for changes. My peace of mind is fragile. It's a risk to invest in my life again; I don't want to experience the pain, for it to be taken away again.

During these times of anxiety and fear I went straight back to 'stage 1' (page 317) and wanted the reassurance of my oncologist to make my world safe again so I could go out into it and live.

The anniversary of my first diagnosis approached and seemed more poignant than others. I tried to communicate this with a Facebook post. A celebration of this day seemed too much, but to avoid it felt wrong. It is firmly implanted on the timeline of my life so I acknowledge this day in my own way and differently each year. I didn't want anyone to rescue me or feel sorry for me. I simply wanted to say how I felt:

"Much as I loathe this date and the days leading up to it, I will acknowledge it. 11 years ago today at 17:51 and 30 weeks pregnant I was diagnosed with cancer for the first time. Lots of good, fun and happy things have happened since then, and I appreciate every second I am well and alive, but there is a sadness around this date and an anxiety of the future which never quite disappears because everything did change forever. Much love to many people in my life, but especially to Bonnie who unknowingly came on that journey with me and gave me reason, hope and strength when it was beyond hideous. Xxxxx"

I was teary all day, the slow, silent, unstoppable, heavy type of tears which fell from my eyes when I engaged with the events and feelings of that day eleven years ago, and the lonely, frightening hours and days which followed.

I listened to the girls talking and laughing with their friends and it sounded like the sweetest sound I had ever heard. I appreciated every single noise they were making and marvelled at what I would have given back then to know that I would be alive eleven years on. What would have occupied my mind for so much of the time instead of those deep dark thoughts of fear and sadness? We went food and school-shoe shopping, and had the house alarm serviced, and the kids bickered, so it was pretty much a normal day, but the sadness hung heavy on and in me. Bonnie seemed to sense this and to lighten the mood sucked her gravy through a straw at teatime, much to the distain of Ian, but it made me laugh and laugh, and again gave me the reminder I needed of how much I was grateful for.

I then headed for the first anniversary of my second cancer diagnosis. I was unsure about how I would feel it. I looked back over the last year. This time last year I didn't even know I had cancer again. I looked back on what I had achieved and been through, and wondered how I survived the physical and emotional aspects of cancer for a second time. This cancerversary feels very different to cancerversary number one, which is full of searing sadness. This for some reason feels strange; how can one person have been through so much and not given up, not crumpled in a corner and said they couldn't go on? I felt proud of what I had achieved and how I had coped with my treatment and recovery over the previous twelve months.

The next six-monthly check-up was looming. As the day approached, time seemed to speed up. I began to think about this time next week, this time in four days, three days, two days, this time tomorrow. Time depleting. Anxiety increasing. Counting down that something might change, health might change; my freedom and choice might change and be ripped away from me in a moment, out of my control and choice. The anxiety was excruciating and for the first time I wanted someone to come with me to the appointment to hold my hand, to support me, to comfort me, to rescue me, to stand in my place of despair and fear with me.

I sat crying in the waiting room with an overwhelming fear of what was going to be found, said, tested or asked. Were my plans for the next twelve months going to be wiped out yet again? I was able to rationalise that I felt well and had no symptoms, but the waves of feelings from the unknown and fear continued to crash over and through me. Nothing could contain the tears of helplessness and fear that fell throughout the appointment. I felt sorry for the registrar who I sat in front of, having to witness me, but I could not contain my feelings any more. My resolve had been weakened and was worn away over time. And then, the relief surging through my mind and body that nothing was found; I was free to carry on, to make arrangements and enjoy life. I left the consultation room feeling I could give myself permission to live the next few months, until the next appointment.

The not such good news was that my oncologist had taken a sabbatical. I felt abandoned and scared without his presence, the secure and safe base we seek when we are frightened or at risk in some way. I bargained that I didn't need him now and would deal with his absence if I needed to.

I look back at the two anniversaries and the check-up. It was a sad and anxious time, which held me back from enjoying the here and now and the future. I felt frustrated that my thoughts were being occupied by cancer for so much of the time; they were holding me back from living. I oscillated between wanting to move on and being stuck where I was. There was so much to work out and understand; cancer is not just a physical illness, it touches every part of our lives. I was trying to work out and understand how cancer had affected me, and attended a short course on self-esteem and body image. During the course there was an exercise where we had to write a letter to our bodies. Here is mine:

"Dear Body

Thank you for being there for me through cancer twice. Thank you for recovering and not giving up twice. I know you have changed, as I have, but we are still together and here alive. Cancer is something that we have been through together. I will look after you because without you I can't do the things that make me feel happy and alive. Thank you body, we are a great team.

Love Mind and Soul xx"

As we shared our letters, I tearily reflected how grateful I was that my body had recovered and that without my body how different my life would be. Rather than reflecting on how it looked and what had changed through age and cancer, I focused instead on what it was able to do. My body allowed me to do the things that gave my life satisfaction, passion and meaning. I will never stop admiring or appreciating my body, and how it coped and recovered, how it overcame the ravages of the treatment for cancer.

The pink fluffy fun stuff started to arrive on shop shelves and in the pages of magazines ahead of Breast Cancer Awareness month in October. My frustration was brewing. Fun and cancer are not words I associate together, and certainly not if you have had a diagnosis of breast cancer or any other type of cancer for that matter. I have done fun things because I have had cancer and have been driven by an insatiable energy to achieve while I can, fuelled by fear of missing out later in life. I've tried to squidge a seventy-five year life into ten, just in case time and health run out for me. My life may look fun from the outside, but it's not fun to live with fear or the possibility of a recurrence happening at any time in any place.

Red hearts, chain emails and social media posts about where you keep your handbag, what colour bra you are wearing, and how many tattoos you have claim to raise awareness, but I'm not sure how. I find these posts insensitive and pointless. I wonder if people consider what level of awareness or involvement they want with cancer in their lives? Do we just want to know there is a disease called cancer, but avoid any further thoughts or feelings? Do we want to post these types of posts and feel absolved from taking any further action or responsibility? Do we want to fundraise or volunteer at a cancer charity? Do we take testing, to discover what our lifetime risk of cancer is, which may give us a temporary reassurance knowing we are disease-free? Do people take their hands and eyes away from their keyboards each year, month, week, day to check their bodies for change? Do we donate to cancer charities? Are we aware of how this money is used? Are we aware of the latest cuts to funding for life-saving and life-extending drugs? That, to me, is awareness. I shared my views on Facebook:

> "I am aware with the anniversaries of two cancer diagnoses in the next few weeks there is the possibility that I am being a tad sensitive, but early detection and better treatments save lives from cancer, not the fluffy pink stuff that is about to descend into inboxes, screens, and the media. Posting a make-up-less selfie, red heart etc. can be fun, but please also make a donation and give yourself the once-over as well, because that is the part that is going to increase the length of a life and maybe your own."

Although my physical health continued to improve and I had worked through my anger, I felt hopeless and depressed without focused goals or objectives. The depression was starting to get to me now. I was filling my day, but not feeling I was achieving. I felt hollow, pointless, worthless and lost. I was beginning to give up. I contemplated going to see my GP about these feelings. I had allowed myself enough time to physically heal and now needed something else. I had played it safe and now I needed a challenge to focus on and work towards, but nothing reckless. And that is how and when my second bucket list was devised, goals and focus to draw me out of this pit of depression and hopelessness.

I was feeling unproductive as I recovered from cancer, feeling well enough to do something but not knowing how much or what to do, and I was stagnating as per 'stage 7' (page 319). I still hadn't found 'meaning' (page 322) to my life after cancer and was searching for this but recognised I had the 'freedom' (page 322) to choose.

My second bucket list:

1. Collect Bonnie on her last day of primary school (what an achievement, to be alive to take her on her first day and to be there to collect her on her last).
2. Choose 10 things to celebrate my 50th birthday: have a tattoo (yes, very mid-life crisis); go to Wimbledon tennis tournament; go skiing with the girls; drive a tractor (carried over from bucket list number one); see Trooping the Colour; trek to Machu Picchu; see inside the Royal Albert Hall; climb Blackdown Hill (a hill I see daily from where I live – I frequently wondered what the reciprocal view would look like); visit Ypres and Buckingham Palace.
3. Promote awareness for better understanding of the experience of cancer (this is how I began to write this book, and it came from my awareness and frustration second time around about how

cancer patients are treated and how little is spoken about the emotional and psychological impact of cancer).

4. See both Poppy and Bonnie into university (I wanted the girls to have interesting careers which would enable them to have jobs they could travel the world with; this stemmed from my regrets about further education and not having a career).

I chose these bucket list items by imagining I was lying on my death bed and thinking about what I would wish I had done and seen, the repeated and yet unsolvable death calculations rumbling in my mind, the unpredictability of life, and yet the certainty of death, ever present. The only way forward is to think about living, living to the full, every single, gorgeous, precious second. This bucket list was more condensed than the last. It had slightly ramped up in urgency, having had cancer twice, but was scaled down in size as I was aware there was probably less time available to me now. I also accepted I can't do everything. I will die not having achieved all I want to and not having seen all that I want to see, but this makes what I do choose more special, because in choosing these I have had to rule other things out.

With hope for the future and goals planned to focus on, my mood improved. I had more energy and fewer aches and pains, and I realised that this was what I needed in my life to create a distraction from cancer and all it may take from me. This felt to be from a different place than the last time, not from a place of fear, anger or rebellion, but from a calmer place, a place of sadness and with some acceptance of the finiteness of time and life, and not wanting regrets when that time comes.

> *Following the mindfulness course, I had less anger and anxiety and my focus had shifted; I wanted to use my time well and feel satisfied at what I had achieved, seen and experienced as per 'stage 8' (page 319). After my physical recovery, my life lacked focus in my 'spiritual' (page 324) dimension and the bucket list provided this.*

I booked the sponsored trek to Machu Picchu for September 2015. Bucket list 2015, item one: tick. I was terrified at the prospect of what I had taken on, so terrified in fact that I told no one for several months. I would have to train and prepare properly for this. What if I'm not fit enough? What if I'm ill there? What if I don't meet anyone I like on the trek? I hated the thought of leaving the girls but also wanted to be a role model to them. A role model of courage, focus and determination, facing and overcoming adversity, going out and exploring this wonderful world we live in, coming back to tell them about my tales of travel, and achieving my goals and helping others. I set myself the target of raising £5,000 for Breast Cancer Care, the charity who had given me so much over the years, the charity which helped me find focus and hope when I was depressed, desperate and hopeless. I wanted to offer something back to those who follow on this journey after me. I wanted to make a difference to breast cancer patients. But what if I failed? What if I couldn't raise the money… the chit-chat rumbled on in my head.

The new vigour was promptly followed by a body failure. I went out walking for what I intended to be a short walk and so wore wellies. It turned into a long walk and because I felt so good, I went out running for the next two days, planning to clock up the Machu Picchu training miles. My left foot began to hurt and then it really hurt. Google informed me that I had broken a metatarsal, and icing and resting it would be a good idea, for the next six weeks. I wouldn't be starting the Machu Picchu trek training any time soon then. One step forward, two steps back.

I partied just about non-stop for six weeks over Christmas 2014, feeling that I was making up for missing out on the last one, saying yes to each and every invitation. The partying took its toll and 2015 began with recovering from the broken foot, a sinus infection and a cycling crash on black ice, putting my training and plans for 2015 on hold further. I avoided any thoughts of failing, training and fundraising, and booked a skiing trip for February half-term – bucket list 2015, item two: tick.

The year 2015 began with mixed feelings. I was nervous of what I had planned, but also excited about the year I was going to be fifty, Poppy was going to become a teenager and Bonnie would be leaving primary school. It was a milestone birthday for me, a milestone year of celebration and achievement. Tentative plans were made for my fiftieth birthday celebrations and trek fundraising. Life felt good, I didn't have the desire to achieve everything yesterday. I took my time and paced myself; I wanted to savour and enjoy each moment, each moment of a year I didn't assume I would be alive for. I was slowly and steadily breaking free from the tether of cancer and beginning to invest in my life again.

It was with a few tears in my eyes that I reflected that I finished my treatment a year ago, and I acknowledged this with a Facebook post:

"A year ago today I finished my cancer treatment. A lot has happened since then and there is still much more to do! A few people have been asking where I am with treatment, so: I have a daily tablet called letrozole (my cancer needs hormones to grow so this stops the cancer and hormones meeting), a monthly implant called goserelin to make sure the letrozole works to the max effect and then, because of years of treatment, I now have osteoporosis so I have an annual infusion called zoladronic acid to strengthen my bones and it also reduces the risk of secondary bone cancer. These meds have caused some weight gain and give me really really stiff and painful joints. I also have an annual mammogram and six-monthly check-ups. I'm here, happy and healthy and that's what counts. xx"

I found offering periodic updates stopped intrusive questions at times when I wanted to focus on other things.

CHAPTER 21

"Your vision will become clear
only when you look into your heart.
Who looks outside, dreams.
Who looks inside, awakens."

Carl Jung

On 14th February after much arranging, packing, purchasing and checking of kit, we went to Pamporovo in Bulgaria for a week's skiing with Poppy and Bonnie. I was so excited to see their faces and share this experience with them. I hadn't skied for twenty years and much had changed in my mind and body in that time. I was nervous of falling and hurting myself, especially with the osteoporosis diagnosis because any breaks or fractures were excluded from my travel insurance cover. Any fracture or breaks would not only be expensive but would also have a massive impact on the training needed for the trip to Machu Picchu;

the consequences would just not be worth it. I no longer loved the adrenalin rush or hurtling down an ice-covered red run at speed, out of control, giggling and screaming with the danger. I now lived with the fear and danger of cancer, and I was happier snow ploughing down a green run having had time to take in the view. I had changed. Poppy, as I had anticipated, was a wonderful skier and within twelve hours of arriving home wanted to return to the slopes, and that season if possible. Bonnie was more cautious and nervous but enjoyed herself.

The trip built my confidence and trust in life again and reduced my 'unfinished business' (page 331).

Each week that passed brought my annual mammogram closer. I was strangely calm as the appointment crept closer. I now knew that this was the easy bit, although physically uncomfortable. Far worse were the psychological issues of the results, waiting and worrying. The next check-up was a couple of weeks away, so I did my best to keep busy and hold my grip of not slip-sliding into the cycle of anxiety and depression that tests and appointments created.

At my six-monthly check I caught a glimpse of my oncologist. I tracked his movements from my waiting room chair at the clinic and I felt like a groupie, hoping to meet their idol. He entered and left consultation rooms, sleeves rolled to his elbow, strong, focused, confident, cool and calm, with an air of well-earned respect surrounding him. It felt reassuring he was back. I didn't expect to see him, but I really wanted to, to show him I was here, happy and, I hoped, healthy, and to thank him for his part in this, for being a rock of safety and voice of calm and hope, the prescriber of treatment and life. I wanted to show him the outcome of his work. I was again strangely calm in the build-up to this appointment as well. I knew I was okay. I felt well and couldn't feel anything that shouldn't be there, having checked repeatedly and microscopically during the preceding days. My instincts were right and after an hour's wait, I had had this confirmed. And breathe, breathe, breathe. Relief, the tension evaporated from my tensed muscles. It was hard to listen to a lady in the waiting room who was crying out in pain at each small movement she made and was a stark reminder of how cancer can progress and how health changes.

With my injuries healed and my check-up and mammogram clear, I could no longer avoid the more focused planning, training and fundraising for Machu Picchu, all of which scared me. But I could avoid them no longer. I had been declared healthy and the fear of failure was looming and becoming the greater fear.

The trek training gained momentum. Short walks first and then longer and then over more difficult terrain, pushing my body a bit more as each week went by, following the training schedule, hours and pounds burnt up along footpaths and tracks. I was beginning to hate the sight of my walking boots and the dog was beginning to hate the sight of me. My sister-in-law was also turning fifty this year and was also undertaking a trek, so we trained together where possible. Some days we had to go with our four children, who moaned like hell and we had to bribe them with Coke and chips to continue up the next hill and around the next corner.

As I trained I began to think about the fundraising side of the trek. I worked through a gazillion ideas: jumble sales, activity days, cake sales, race nights, dress-down days at work. It seemed a lot to organise and manage when time was already a precious commodity. After much discussing and pondering we decided to hold one large event, attempting to raise the money in one go. 'Bex's Black Tie Ball' was crafted and was to be held in early September. We looked at venues and menus, and we planned ticket prices and entertainment. We had a logo and invitation designed, set up Facebook and Just Giving pages, created Excel spreadsheets to keep track of costs, and started promoting sales. We asked family and friends for their support, and contacted local businesses to source prizes for the raffle and lots for the auction. It was hard work and required continuous motivation and drive in the face of setbacks, let downs and rejections, revising plans and asking for help. Interest began to build and I was touched with the support, kindness and generosity of people. We had donations for meals and boxes of wine from local pubs, a car valet, a weekend in a cottage, a guided walk on the South Downs, a drive in a vintage car and a drive in a sports car. I promoted the prizes, the evening and the cause relentlessly.

Trek training continued to gain momentum and, much to my delight, I was finally losing the treatment and menopause weight gain. Result. At times I was SO bored with the hours of walking that I wanted to scream, but I kept going. I could almost crack walnuts with my thighs they were so strong, pillars of steel that kept me upright and going. I became toned and tanned, loving the focus the training provided. I could shut out my fears about dying and replace them with miles, views, big pieces of sugary flapjack and the burning of calories.

The ball plans and arrangements progressed, until I asked for payment, at which point several people cancelled. Several people cancelled whole tables. I felt let down. I smiled and replied sweetly, but couldn't help but think I hope they are never in the position of needing the support of Breast Cancer Care, or even mine. I was panicking and felt well out of my comfort zone with what I had taken on. I started a more focused campaign to sell the remaining tickets and pushed myself to be pushy, which goes against the grain of who I am. I wished I didn't care so much about getting things right and being a perfectionist.

As April changed into May, I started to get excited about my birthday. I could not believe I was going to be fifty. Who would have thought, dared, imagined that I would still be here twelve years and two cancers later? Celebratory plans were made and shopping trips taken. I loved waking up to see boxes of prosecco, party dresses and elegant high heels dotted around my bedroom. I took a break from the trek training, as I wanted to enjoy every single moment of my birthday and my birthday month. I will have lived with cancer in my thirties, forties and now fifties and I am proud of that. I hope I can inspire hope in others who face a similar diagnosis, to live their lives fully, to thrive in adversity.

Lovely Brother arrived from Sydney for a schoolmate's wedding and it conveniently coincided with my ten days of birthday celebrations, which felt like a middle-class '18–30s Holiday'. We started off with a massive house party, complete with DJ, photo booth, helium balloons and cocktail bar.

Next up was a comedy show and dinner, an afternoon tea party and climbing the O2 to enjoy spectacular views of London. All too soon we were heading back to Terminal 3 departures for another teary goodbye. It was a fantastic ten days and great to celebrate in so many different ways with so many people. I felt truly loved. I thought back to how I felt that time last year and how I never thought I would feel happy or be able to enjoy life, and that the paralysing fear would never leave me, but it had.

Bonnie was leaving primary school in July and for the whole academic year I had been thinking, at each event and milestone which forms part of the ritual of the year, that this would be the last. There was a sadness to these; the last autumn term arriving with shiny new shoes and lunch box, the last Christmas Fayre, the last school play, the last parent's evening, the last school trip, the last packed lunch, the last newsletter, the last school run; events which I didn't think I would be here for when my life changed on 19th August 2003 at 17:51.

The trigger for my grief was Bonnie's last sports day at primary school: a traditional day of fun and competitive banter; children wearing their house team colours and parents whooping and cheering as streaks of colour and focused faces ran along the chair-lined track; lanes marked out in chalky white; a picnic of refined sugar, e-numbers, and sneaky bottles of wine consumed on rugs spread out like patchwork quilts on a freshly mowed field in the summer sunshine; the laughter, the banter and – this year – the tears hidden behind smiles and sunglasses. I had thought I was doing okay, emotionally, about her ending primary school, excited about her taking the next step into secondary school and relief at having two children with the same uniform, school times and inset days. But I wasn't.

I was teary as Bonnie ran her races and competed in her field events. I didn't care if she was first or last. I had another focus, maybe a focus which others take for granted. Quite simply, I was there. I was watching my world, my hopes, my dreams, dressed in a yellow t-shirt with her long blonde hair blowing in the summer breeze, smiling with her friends. My world was running down the track, my world hurling bean bags, my world jumping horizontally and then vertically, my world with her long spindly legs and flat feet, my world in a grubby crumpled t-shirt that should probably have been freshly ironed for this special day. My world was alive. My eyes never left my world that day.

I was proud that the little baby who had had such a risky start to life was healthy and happy, and had no recollection of what she had been through. I felt guilty about what I had put her through, what I gave her no choice in. I had put all of this at risk for her. This could all have been so very different. I now knew that the next few weeks of leavers' ceremonies were going to be emotional because I realised how far we had both come, how much we had both achieved and the people we had become both together and apart; two halves of a story, one half with no recollection and one half who carried the burden of guilt and pain.

I was crying for the days that I didn't think I would have. I was crying because I wanted to be well enough to take Bonnie to school on her first day and there I was, likely to be well enough to be there to collect her on her last. I was crying because I hadn't had to die publicly and be the pitied playground victim and gossiped about. I was crying because I had protected Bonnie from that. I was crying because I had achieved my goal and well beyond. I was crying because I was grieving. I was letting go of how hard it had been to stay focused, to keep going, to keep smiling, to keep inspiring, to keep achieving, to keep living with the fear.

As I headed into Bonnie's last few days at primary school, the grief and the tears increased and intensified. So other people knew what was going on, I posted this on Facebook:

"The end of Year 6 will mean something different to us all and our little darlings. For me it is relief and pride at being Bonnie's mum and that I am here to do that when so many times I nearly wasn't, even before she was born. I spent five years wishing and hoping I would be alive to take her to school on her first day at primary school, that was enough for me, thankfully I am alive on her last. I haven't always enjoyed being a mum but I have appreciated it. Basically I'm going to be crying about this a lot this week so just ignore me! Xxx"

The last day of the school year is steeped in rituals, providing a framework for the ending to take place in. The day begins with an assembly in which each Year 6 child takes a part. There were songs, poems, gym displays, comedy sketches and thank yous. There were photos, achievements and a million memories from the last seven years: of small, anxious, shy children dressed in large clothes, to pre-teens, confident and sassy, ready to take the next step in their lives. And then someone started crying. It rapidly became like a dominoes game, and soon children, parents and teachers were crying and once we started we couldn't stop. Tears fell, hugs were given and photos were taken to capture every precious last second. The assembly ended with a quote I had not heard before and it has stayed with me: "*Don't cry because it's over, smile because it happened*" from the film Dr Seuss. How very true.

The end of the academic year is marked with the children who are leaving passing through an arch formed by the children who are not. We reluctantly left the playground for the last time, this was the end. The end of something I had barely hoped that I would see the first day of, let alone the last. The tears and the depression about this ending persisted for weeks and I began to accept that this day, much like the day of diagnosis, was always going to reduce me to tears when I thought about it because it meant so much to me.

These were events that I appreciated being alive to see because they might not have happened. They built on making me feel safe again, as per 'stage 1' (page 317), and I felt connected in my 'social' (page 323) and 'personal' (page 324) dimensions.

CHAPTER 22

"In the end, just three things matter:
How well we have lived,
how well we have loved
and how well we have learned to let go."

Jack Kornfield

The logistics of the ball, trek training, summer holidays, work, teens and pre-teens were starting to take their toll. It felt relentless and exhausting. There was so much to arrange and rearrange. There was a permanent and growing to-do list and people changing their minds and then changing their minds again. I am an organised person and last-minute changing of anything is not my cup of tea. Calm not chaos. Planned not spontaneous. My mind was whirring at speed twenty-four seven.

The cycle of anniversaries and emotions clicked onto repeat as 19th August arrived once more. Ball and trek mania kept me distracted, until the day when I woke crying, silent and heavy tears which needed to fall, tears which could not be resolved or removed. Ian gave me a massive hug and just held me in his arms as I silently did what I needed to do. Today would be a makeup-less day of sobs and smiles. It was the last day of a break we took in Dorset and looking at Bonnie playing so innocently in a rubber dingy splashing around in a lagoon reminded me I was so glad to be alive, so glad to be her mum and so glad that she knew nothing of how shit it all had been. I wonder how many other people wake up on a day that changed their life like this; the day death arrives in your life, a fact that you can't ever really forget or move away from once you start thinking about it.

A few days later I set off with Poppy and Bonnie to London for Buckingham Palace State Rooms and Gardens tour, another 2015 bucket list item. London was busy and it was raining but nothing spoiled my mood. To the embarrassment of Poppy and Bonnie I 'oohhed' and 'ahhhed' my way through the magnificent splendour; long rooms filled with historic art, ornately decorated ceilings and acres and acres of sumptuous fabrics adorning walls, windows and furniture. There was gilt and crystal everywhere, creating flashes of sparkle as they caught the light. We ate cake and drank tea in the palace garden afterwards, relaxing in the pristine and iconic surroundings, the noise of London around us.

And with a slight morning chill in the air, we moved into September, a busy month of landmark occasions and anniversaries. Bonnie began secondary school, a day of emotion, excitement and relief. I was proud I was there, fit and well, to witness her beginning the next chapter of her life, a beginning which I appreciated being a part of, relieved I had witnessed another milestone. I was also relieved Poppy was there to help her if she needed, a surrogate protector until she found her way.

The ball to-do list reached what felt like epic and overwhelming proportions, and I found it hard to focus on anything. This was tough, as everyone else seemed so excited and I wanted to share their excitement, but I was consumed by my fear. The Just Giving donations came rolling in and I was touched by people's support and generosity.

I had written a speech, which I hoped would provide a heartfelt insight of what it was like to have cancer. I couldn't say the speech without crying, no matter how many times I rehearsed. I couldn't detach from the emotion it generated, but I didn't want to detract from the honesty it was written with, so if I cried on the night, I cried. I ticked the days off, and the tasks kept on growing. My patience was low and was being consumed by the ball. I was short-tempered and didn't think I was being such a good role model or mother to Poppy and Bonnie.

Ball day arrived. The schedule and tasks were well-rehearsed in my head. I was reliant on so many people helping out with so many things, I couldn't keep track of them all. I felt paralysed with anxiety. People were still changing things. I kept juggling and adjusting to keep up. I tried to stay calm and focused on the goal, providing people with a great night and to raise the fundraising target. It felt a big responsibility that was resting firmly and precariously on my shoulders.

We arrived early afternoon at the venue, en masse, and began to decorate the room. We began blowing up balloons with a huge helium cylinder and tied them with ribbon. The white, light and airy room, which overlooked a perfectly manicured lush green golf course, became transformed with the eye-catching Breast Cancer Care logo colours of fuchsia pink and vibrant orange. Glass shone and cutlery clinked. We set up further tables with themed sweets to sell, collection boxes were dotted around the room and we placed literature about the services and work that Breast Cancer Care provide on each table. And breathe.

Home for a quick shower, clothes changed, make-up applied, perfume sprayed, hair blow-dried and we returned to the venue. I held up my long dress as we walked across the gravel car park. My mouth was dry and my heart pumping faster, fuelled by adrenalin. Poppy and Bonnie looked different with their plaited hair, out of their trainers and leggings and in dresses and shoes. They looked utterly gorgeous.

I was still being bombarded with last-minute changes and tweaking, questions and decisions. People began to arrive. Each and every one was greeted and thanked by me, grateful and humbled by their support; gorgeous girls in high heels and stunning dresses, and dapper boys, smart in their crisp white shirts and shiny shoes. The room began to fill with smiling faces, laughter and atmosphere. Prosecco was poured and photographs were taken. The evening began to gather pace.

We sat for the starter. I could hardly eat; my speech was next on the printed and published running order. There was no escape. Face your fears. I drank two vodkas at speed. I felt marginally better. I hate crowds and I hate attention and public speaking is my nemesis, and now all three were about to come together. I hoped this wouldn't end badly. Maybe just one more shot of vodka. Maybe not. I had to do this; I had to overcome these fears to achieve my goal to raise awareness, to change something for someone somewhere. The speech was heartfelt and emotional and now I had to deliver it to the 132 faces in front of me. Gulp. Breathe. Gulp. I could feel the love and support in the room for me urging me on as I made my way to the front. I turned and was blinded by the bright lights. I shuffled my papers and focused on the words in front of me. Go, Bex, go. The words on the pages entered the room by my shaky voice and the room fell still and silent.

I made my way through the words and pages; my story, and how Breast Cancer Care and their forum had saved my mind. And then at the end people were standing and clapping and crying. I had done it. I had spoken about my inner fears and given insight of what it is like to have cancer. Not once did I use the words 'brave', 'fight' and 'strong', because people who have had cancer talk about cancer differently to the sensationalist headlines printed in the media. I returned to my seat. I could breathe again.

Here is a part of the speech:

"Hello, I will try to do this without crying or being sick or, worst case scenario, both!

Firstly, thank you from the bottom of my heart for coming along this evening to support me and Breast Cancer Care. Without your kindness and generosity this event wouldn't be happening. Every penny you spend here tonight (with the exception of the bar!) will be going directly to Breast Cancer Care. Thank you also to those who have donated to the raffle and auction to create a quality, and possibly the most eclectic, list of donations ever.

Being diagnosed and living with cancer isn't just about the physical aspect, there are also the emotional and physiological aspects too. Being diagnosed with cancer is rubbish, being treated for cancer is rubbish, living with cancer is rubbish and watching some with cancer is no doubt rubbish too. And speaking from experience, being diagnosed with cancer when pregnant is particularly rubbish.

I was first diagnosed with breast cancer twelve years ago when I was thirty weeks pregnant with Bonnie. Chemo was offered that afternoon by my oncologist (who I am still totally in love with). A year's worth of treatment followed. Ten years later and ironically in the appointment that my oncologist was going to discharge me, I was diagnosed with a recurrence of a similar cancer in the lymph nodes above my collar bone, my long-term survival isn't great.

I went to hell and back on more than one occasion. Cancer is isolating, cancer is full of unknown, cancer is full of uncertainty, cancer is full of waiting, cancer is full of difficult conversations and choices, followed by more waiting. This all set on a back drop of fear. Fear of dying, fear of the treatment not working, fear was this going to be my last birthday, Christmas, Mother's Day? And my biggest fear of them all, the fear of saying goodbye to Poppy and Bonnie.

Cancer never quite goes away. The moment you are diagnosed with cancer everything you know, planned, hoped and dreamed about changes. Cancer affected every part of my life, my heart and my soul. It destroyed who I thought I was and where I thought I was going.

In time, from the decimation came a small shoot of hope. And that small shoot of hope was Breast Cancer Care. I stumbled upon their online chat room during a random Googling session about survival statistics. Four hours later I was still there. The online chat room was perfect for me, I could be an anonymous voyeur and have access twenty-four hours a day. I was wowed by the stories I read and felt connected and less isolated. I wasn't the only young mum struggling and scared. In time, I moved from reading to posting, and in a bit more time I was supporting others who had just begun their rubbishness of cancer. This was the beginning of who I was going to become and am today.

Bit by bit, and super slowly, the fear and despair lessened and were replaced with a passion for life and a hope to help people who face a similar diagnosis. The fear is now harnessed and adds a very sharp sense of focus to my life, because life is short and I don't take for granted that I will be healthy tomorrow.

What I liked about Breast Cancer Care was the space and freedom to talk openly and eventually use my experience of cancer; this is deeply cathartic on a personal level and, I hope, inspirational and comforting to others. So, as my oncologist saved my life physically, Breast Cancer Care saved me emotionally and psychologically.

Sadly millions more women – our friends, sisters, wives, mothers and daughters – are going to be diagnosed with breast cancer. I hope tonight we can make a difference to them so they find the support they need.

So, when I reach Machu Picchu with my thighs of steel and a big grin on my face, and no doubt a tear in my eye, I will raise a glass to you all."

The main course, raffle, dessert, auction and DJ followed into the night. As darkness fell outside, twinkly lights lit the room and laughter filled the sombre silence of earlier. Money was being raised for someone somewhere who will hear the words 'you have breast cancer'; someone with a name and a treatment plan, someone who was as shocked and as scared as me. We will never meet, we will never know each other's faces or names or share our treatment regimes, but we will have shared so much. We will both know what those words sound like and mean and the effect they have on our lives and those in our lives.

The evening was an extraordinary success and exceeded all of my expectations, an evening where £10,000 was raised for Breast Cancer Care, an evening which began because one tiny cell in my body didn't do what it should have done. Many thank yous were made over the coming days to everyone who supported the event in so many ways.

I was finding it hard to connect with what I had achieved, and to hear and read the comments about the evening and my speech. I seemed to have touched people; a story of sadness and disaster followed by hope and triumph, conquering adversity, living a life. I reflected that this crazy idea of trekking to Machu Picchu to raise £5,000 for Breast Cancer Care was dreamt up when I had felt hopeless and depressed, and that idea had given me a focus, something to plan and live for, to ignite my desire to move on and live again. The idea and the achievement were a year apart, and the feelings were two people apart. One was so depressed and hopeless she could hardly be arsed to get out of bed, and the other – trim, fit, focused and living her life.

I'm using less counselling theory to describe my experience now, as I understand what I have been through and where to place cancer in my life. I have learnt of the finiteness of time and to use my time well, which gives my life increased 'meaning' (page 322) and gives fulfilment in my 'social' (323), 'personal' (page 324) and 'spiritual' (page 324) dimensions. This has reduced my 'anger' (page 326) and anxiety at what changed and was 'out of control' (page 333), and the 'unfinished business' (page 331) in my life.

CHAPTER 23

"Walk as if you are kissing the Earth with your feet."

Thich Nhat Hanh

Cancerversary number two, year two, followed the high of the ball. Cancerversary number one has come to represent the sadness of all that was taken and lost, whereas cancerversary number two has become a celebration of all that I have achieved, and that ball was some achievement.

My mind has attached different meanings to my cancerversaries; one full of loss and sadness, and one full of celebration and achievement. This allows a time and a place to acknowledge and express the feelings cancer has created for me.

Then came check-up day. I had faced my fears with the ball and I was now facing more. I woke up anxious and this continued to build until I cried with fear. I had performed the same check day after day, and felt fit, well and healthy, and there were no signs, no symptoms, no lumps or bumps. But… what if they find something? Something I don't know about. I felt out of control and scared. When I arrived at the hospital I couldn't focus on what I had brought to read to distract myself. The words could not hold my attention. I was vaguely amused and also irritated by the man who was moaning about his appointment being fifteen minutes late. 'Look at the bigger picture' I wanted to say – free healthcare, and life and death.

The big white board in the waiting room informed me that I was waiting in my oncologist's clinic. As I looked more closely, an additional word had been added next to his name. 'Retired'. Fuck. A flood of thoughts and emotions entered my head all at once. I was sad and now more scared; he was my big safe rock in all of the ocean of cancer crap. He had fought my corner and I didn't know if I could trust another oncologist like I trusted him. I felt sad I hadn't been able to say goodbye to someone who had played such a significant part in my life, to say one last thank you and tell him any of this: that he had saved my life, that he had given me time with my children, that he had given me time to make so many memories and achieve so much. But I was also happy for him and hoped he was enjoying a long, happy, healthy and very well-deserved retirement. I was one of thousands of patients he had treated. He was the one person, out of thousands in my life, who saved me. That will always be special. I hope he reads this book. I was left feeling bereft, knowing he was no longer my oncologist and that this was how I had found out, reading the word 'retired' on a noticeboard in a waiting room with a man moaning about waiting, seated on a grotty grey plastic chair surrounded by tatty magazines.

I grieved the loss of my oncologist over the coming months. He had given me hope that I could reach the next goal, and the next milestone, and had played an inspiring and vital role in my life. I had used the hope, and converted it into motivation and actions to live while I could. My oncologist was like no other doctor I had ever met. He saw beyond the illness to me as a person and what I needed to get through the treatment and recovery and to learn to live again on the other side. He engaged with me and stepped into my world, my world of fear and desperation. He adapted his consultation to what I needed. He carefully offered evidence-based facts, balanced with my needs and values. His passion for giving me the best opportunity for life was clear to see and feel.

The check-up was fine and I left feeling I had permission to go to Machu Picchu and trek the Inca Trail, free from worry and an imminent cancer return. Like the cancerversaries and check-ups, Bonnie's birthday celebrations came round once again, a happy time with the customary three rounds of cakes, candles, cards and celebrations. Once these milestones had passed I felt free to begin the trek kit collection in earnest. It felt like a marathon just getting the kit together; what do you wear on a night out in Cusco??? We seemed to need everything from a bikini to a snow jacket. Water bottles, a medical kit, ice packs; I now wonder if it would have been a good idea to have had the rabies' jabs in case I got bitten by a stray dog?

Trek departure day arrived: a day of packing, repacking and managing hopes and nerves. I finally crammed all the kit into an oversized and overweight suitcase and headed off to Terminal 2 to meet my fellow trekkers.

We arrived in Cusco one night and three flights later, a stunning city high in altitude and low on oxygen. Unfortunately not all our suitcases made it onto the second and therefore third flight, and mine was one of them. I now wished I had packed my hand luggage more thoughtfully and not just jammed in what didn't fit in my suitcase, because I didn't actually need a travel towel or bikini just now. Thankfully I had worn my walking boots so could take part in the first two altitude acclimatisation walks in and around Cusco. We borrowed underwear and toiletries, and laughed at our misfortune. It was tough, however. I felt out of my comfort zone and away from all that was familiar and safe. I missed my possessions; they were all I had that was familiar in this unfamiliar land. Our missing luggage finally arrived twenty-eight hours late and just in time for us to repack our kit into four bags which we would see at various points in the trek.

I met my room and tent mate for the trip. We were both down to earth and liked laughing and silence in equal quantities. We shared tales of travelling and snippets of our lives late into the night. When l would get stressed at not being able to find my possessions, she would calmly say 'look with your eyes and not your mouth', and I now say that to my children. One of my all-time favourite photos was taken of us laughing and looking pretty awful outside our tent early one morning with the mountains standing tall in the back ground.

There were twenty-two of us on the trip, plus two guides, a doctor, a kitchen team and porters. We gradually got to know each other over bus rides, meals and the walking. We were a mix of ages, nationalities, backgrounds and careers; some assertive and domineering, some soft and passive, and allegiances and alliances formed within the group. I could write another book about the group dynamics that evolved but I won't; let's just say I did meet some lifelong friends and there were also some post-trek Facebook deletes and blocks!

The lack of oxygen was hard going and I suffered with heart palpitations and a banging headache if I moved at more than one mile an hour. Many aspirin were consumed along the way to help with the headaches. The setting, landscapes, architecture, food and people were mesmerising, as was the night sky, which I saw frequently due to insomnia caused by drinking coca tea to combat the symptoms of being at a high altitude.

After several briefings, we rose early to set off from Cusco to a town where the trek would begin; a six-hour drive away. I was both excited and scared. I checked again that each item was in the right bag. We set off in the darkness and into the unknown. There would be no showers or flushing toilets, no phone signal or internet connection, no mirrors, beds or pillows. Would I be warm enough? Would I need my mascara in bag two or three? Not being a good traveller, I sat at the front of the bus next to a lovely lady whose realness kept me grounded when I started to wobble. We travelled through barren mountain ranges and lush green valleys, through villages, past markets selling donkey heads covered in flies. We drove along narrow roads close to unfenced sheer drops to valleys thousands of feet below us, blind bends galore, and we passed grazing llamas and women bent over carrying firewood on their backs. I savoured every sight and sound. I had worked hard for this. People had donated and supported me generously for this. This was my dream come true, the 'fuck you cancer' trek.

We stopped a few hours later for a delicious lunch prepared from the magic tent perched on the side of the mountain. The crew worked tirelessly throughout the trek, magicking up all sorts of delightful food from seemingly nothing. We had our final briefing, refilled our water bottles and checked our boot laces. This was it, we were off, walking poles in our hands and rucksacks on our backs, excitement in our hearts.

We formed a long line, single file as we joined the track. Soon the pace we were individually comfortable with became apparent and the line became long and broken. We chatted to those in front and behind us. I was used to walking at least three times as fast as this, but I would develop an instant headache if I walked any faster, due to the altitude and reduction of oxygen. My pace was now set by my pounding temples.

We walked slowly through the changing landscape, passing foraging alpacas and Peruvian people, their ruddy cheeks and brightly coloured clothes contrasting with the grey, brown and green land that surrounded them. Children would stop us for photos in exchange for a piece of fruit.

It was tough going and this was only day one, and a half-day trek. Once we reached our camp for the night, there was no climbing into a warm bubble-filled bath, donning my PJs, chatting with my family, updating Facebook with my mileage walked and calories burnt and relaxing in front of the TV, as I had done after my training treks. It was cold and dark and there was little comfort offered from the thin camping mattress. We ate and snuggled down for the night. It was freezing and I slept badly, feeling alone and tearful.

The next day began at 06:30 when the support team brought a bowl of warm water to wash in and a hot drink to our tent. The thought of getting out of my warm sleeping bag and changing my clothes was unpleasant and I undertook this task as quickly as I could, ensuring as little flesh as possible was exposed to the bitter coldness at any one time. We ran, dressed in several layers, to the magic tent, which provided breakfast and the most delicious hot chocolate, before we gathered our rucksacks and poles and headed off for day two of the trek. As we left camp we could not see the summit from the vast valley that lay around, ahead and above us, or the invisible trails which would lead us there. We began to ascend very slowly in the cold, bright air, the sun's rays fiercely strong and clouds rushing past us in the gusting winds. It felt an impossible task and we spread out in a long line, finding again our pace and place within the group. The trails were made of stones of various sizes; it was easy to slip and fall on the unstable narrow trail and I stared at my feet step by step. We paused frequently to gather our breath and look at the views.

Just before lunch we reached the highest point in the trek, an enormous 4,400 metres above sea level, where our trek leader performed a ceremony thanking the gods for getting us to this point. It was moving to watch him. We took plenty of celebratory photographs before we began our descent to the magic tent on a plateau below, which contained our next meal and a welcome sit down.

The trek required both mental and physical stamina, and concentration to keep going despite the discomfort of the altitude and terrain. We chatted away, reminding ourselves why we were doing the trek, the people who we were helping and the people who had helped us get here.

After lunch we walked along the rest of the plateau and began our descent into Huacahuasi, weaving our way along rocky trails, inching ever nearer; children playing football, and goats grazing on the plateau below, which was encircled by a glistening river. I could see the camp already set up with its ordered rows of tents. It was mind-blowingly different and stunningly beautiful. However, I trailed further and further behind in the group, and found it hard to concentrate and motivate myself, which was most unlike me.

As we entered the night's camp, we grabbed our bags and a tent, looking forward to a wash and a rest. The altitude had really affected me and I was teary and worried about the next day, which was nine hours of trekking. I had struggled with the four yesterday and six today. Once we had all arrived, the trek leader asked us to gather round, and he notified us that due to a forty-eight-hour national strike starting in just eight hours' time, the trek itinerary was about to change significantly and immediately. The country would shut down and the roads would be blockaded. If we didn't leave in the next few hours we would be marooned on this stunning plateau and not reach Machu Picchu at all. We had no choice. The porters began dismantling the camp around us as we stood, dazed, trying to work out what we had just heard.

The itinerary, which we had trained and planned for so meticulously, was about to be replaced without notice or choice, and we were going to miss two days of the trek. I was gutted and so was everyone else. I was also feeling guilty because I had been sponsored to do the trek, not to be driven in a minibus. We gathered our possessions and reluctantly boarded the bus once more. We began driving through dusk and then night, the drivers chewing on coca leaves to keep them alert in the darkness. We arrived in the very early morning to a tropical-feeling Ollantaytambo, which was at a much lower altitude. Once more we made our way to our tents, scrabbling around in the darkness.

The next day there was an early morning meeting to decide what to do. The details of the strike were sketchy, and phone calls were made in several languages to several places for the latest news. Plans were made and re-made. We waited for updates and an itinerary, pacing the camp to pass the time. Frustration began to brew, personalities changed. Muttered conversations took place in small groups. Mount Veronica watched, silent and still in the distance, her summit snowy. Eventually two groups formed; a divide, a rift. Some went trekking into the mountains and some went on a historical walk followed by their first freshly ground latte in three days. We met again later and whiled away the evening with card games, eating chicken casserole and chocolate mousse from the magic tent and waiting for news and a plan.

The uncertainty was difficult. I had invested a great deal in this trip. Today we should have had our first sighting of Machu Picchu via the iconic Sun Gate, descending to stay in a hotel in Machu Picchu town with hot running water, a hairdryer and power points. But we weren't; we were wasting time, waiting for a plan. Mount Veronica watched the chaos below her, snowy, stoic, silent and still. The rifts in the group continued and the magic tent kept producing magic three times a day. We waited, wandered and wondered. I held onto the fact that somehow they would get us to Machu Picchu; not getting there would be too awful to even contemplate. Eventually the strike ended and a plan was made. We would be going to Machu Picchu the next day. A peacefulness fell across the camp, although relationships remained changed and strained.

We rose early, dressing in our chosen charity tops. I was so proud to represent Breast Cancer Care. Excitedly we boarded a packed early morning train which would take us to the town of Machu Picchu, from which we would board a bus up to the site. I found my seat, Seat 4, my favourite number. That was special. One of my fellow trekkers gave me a Coke bottle which had my name on it, that was special too. I casually rotated the bottle and noticed the expiry date was Bonnie's birthday. What was going on? Coincidences? Signs? The train pulled slowly out of the station and I felt happy to be finally on my way to Machu Picchu, but sad we had missed so much of the trip. The single train track followed a fast-running winding river just below us. I sat in silence, taking in the views and thinking about the journey I'd been on to get here, arriving at the bustling town of Machu Picchu an hour later.

We walked through a busy market full of souvenirs and joined a long bus queue. It was hot and there wasn't much

British queuing to be seen. We jostled to keep our places. Time was precious. Time was ticking and every moment we spent in the queue was a moment less at Machu Picchu. We boarded the bus and I felt impatient as we made our way up another unfenced vertical mountainside. We disembarked from the bus; it was stiflingly hot and there were swarms of biting mosquitos, but my eyes were drawn to the swallows diving and swooping above our heads. My favourite birds were here, as if to greet me, to welcome me to this goal which had motivated me to live again. I noticed some of the group were wearing tops provided by the trip organiser and my mouth fell open when I read the words surrounding the logo: 'Inspire, Achieve and Believe', the values of Poppy and Bonnie's primary school. The words, the seat number, the Coke bottle and the swallows were poignant moments for me on a poignant day.

We queued for this and we queued for that, slowly getting nearer the views we had planned, trained for and imagined. And then we were there, we were seeing those views, the enormity, the magnificence, the significance, the beauty, the history, the architecture and the intricacies and precision of the masonry. We were given a fascinating talk about Machu Picchu and Inca life as we sat on the terraces where crops would have been grown centuries ago. Sadly we only had a couple of hours at the site and dispersed quickly to see what we wanted to see. I remained on the main site, taking in the history, watching the swallows and the beauty of the valleys below us and the mountains around us, imagining life here all those centuries ago.

All too soon we had to leave Machu Picchu and make our way back down to the town to have lunch and catch the train back to Ollantaytambo, to catch a bus back to Cusco, to have our farewell medal-giving dinner and then repack the four bags into one before catching our flights back to the UK the next day. Only it didn't quite work out like that.

A celebratory lunch, thunderstorm and a couple of cocktails later, we arrived at the station, which was heaving with people waiting everywhere. Our guide began asking questions and making phone calls; a train had derailed further up the single track line. We weren't going anywhere anytime soon. It had already been a long day and now looked like being a lot longer. We sat where we had stood as the sun set. It was then we heard about a plane crash at Cusco Airport. The airport was shut until a plane could be removed from the runway. We waited and waited and waited. We waited five hours for a train in a heaving hall, not daring to move in case we were called to board. We had been up since 5am and the thought of a train journey followed by a bus journey was not the ending I had been hoping for. The farewell medal-giving dinner was struck from the agenda. Eventually we boarded the train and then boarded the bus, arriving in Cusco at 2am. I felt disorientated and sick and went straight to bed. There was still no news about our departure in ten hours' time.

We rose early to make the most of the few remaining hours in Cusco, taking our final walk around the streets, markets and squares before heading to the airport to catch the first of three flights back to the UK. Although we had arrived in good time our seats had been given away and we began a two-hour airport floor wait. I was so bored with waiting. The flight was then delayed and each minute increased our risk of missing the connecting and crucial second flight from Lima to Colombo. We eventually boarded the plane and remained hopeful. The minutes ticked by. By the time we took off we would have about twenty-nine minutes from flight one landing to flight two departing. Despite promises from the airline, supported by the issuing of boarding cards, they did not hold the flight for us and we began a twenty-eight-hour stopover in Lima. I began crying; I felt guilty at impacting further on Ian, I was tired, I was missing the girls and I just wanted to get home. The airline and trip organiser were less than helpful in getting us home; I guess for them it's about the bottom line on a spreadsheet, the line between profit and loss. My line was different; it was about having a hug with my children and ticking a bucket list experience.

Three airports, three countries, two flights and several time zones later, we landed at Heathrow Terminal 5. I rushed through arrivals and customs to see Poppy and Bonnie as soon as possible. I said my goodbyes to my fellow trekkers with tears in my eyes, reminiscing about the adventure which had taken place. We each had a reason to go, a story to tell and memories to take home, and many laughs through the adversity and the achievement.

Machu Picchu was an experience I will always treasure. It gave me hope, focus and purpose, the planning and training forcing me out of a place of hopelessness and depression. Machu Picchu gave me something to work for and to achieve, a distraction from the trauma and destruction cancer had left in its wake, something to force me back to engaging with life once more.

Although the trip was challenging it continued to build my self-esteem as per 'stage 4' (page 318). I had less fear about the finiteness of life because I had less 'unfinished business' (page 331) and had achieved more of my goals as in 'stage 8' (page 319). I felt I had used my time productively and had 'freedom' (page 322) to create 'meaning' (page 322) in my life.

CHAPTER 24

*"Go forward in life with a twinkle in your eye
and a smile on your face, but with great purpose in heart."*

Gordon B. Hinckley

found it hard to adjust to life after the ball and trek, they had been my focus for so long. I drifted unoccupied. What would I do with my time, thoughts and feelings now? The trek and the fundraising had taken a lot out of me physically and I knew I needed to rest and recoup, to take a step back into the shadows. The year 2016 would be about something else; I wanted to enjoy and support the goals and plans of my friends who had supported me in mine. I began to think about the 2016 bucket list. It was small and simple, nothing that was going to take hours of my time, focus or energy: to see Coldplay in concert, to run 5km, try yoga, to watch twelve films and read twelve books. There was a walk I had done many times during the trek training and I had always turned left at the same point, and wondered what it would be like to turn right.

As 2015 drew to a close, I was sad it was ending. I appreciated being here to be able to do each and every one of those amazing things. I didn't take the time or the opportunity for granted: the year I turned fifty, the year Bonnie left primary school, the year I raised £10,000 for a charity, which changed my life. Cancer and I were done, or so I thought.

Cancer doesn't follow the thoughts and hopes we have in our minds. Cancer doesn't think, 'Oh she's had two goes already, I'll move on to someone else'. No, cancer does its own thing wherever and whenever it likes.

A small flesh-coloured raised patch came up seemingly overnight on the side of my face in May 2015. I'd poked and prodded it and it had no suspicious features, so I looked and checked every now and again, and did nothing about it. Casually scrolling through a Facebook feed one evening, I noticed a post shared by a friend about Hugh Jackman who'd had a basal cell carcinoma removed. I had no idea what a basal carcinoma looked like, so I Googled it out of curiosity. Shit, crap and fucking fuck. The images on my screen reflected exactly what was on my face. The next morning I dialled the GP's number repeatedly from two phones until I got through and was able to make an appointment. GP appointment attended. Symptoms described and shown to GP. GP rummaged for a bright lighty thing from his desk drawer and shone it on my face. My eyes winced in the strong beam of white light. I was diagnosed there and then with a basal cell carcinoma, instantly and calmly. Unpleasant but familiar feelings of guilt and anxiety began churning in my abdomen.

While I was there, I also asked about a small red patch which had come and gone on my chest for several years. Sometimes it was itchy and red. Sometimes it was smooth and pink. I had applied hydrocortisone cream during the itchy and red times, and the itch and redness would disappear and then some time later would reappear. The itch and the redness had appeared again in December 2015, and this time, despite the liberal application of the hydrocortisone cream, the itch and the red hadn't disappeared. Bright lighty thing was being shone at this now, and GP said it was currently nothing, but 1 in 1,000 turned into something nasty, so it was added to the referral sheet too. By 09:00 on that February morning, I had been diagnosed with skin cancer. Our marvellous NHS called a couple of hours later and I was offered an appointment with a dermatologist in four days' time. The anxiety and fear came and went. I felt a failure; how could I have been diagnosed with cancer again? One. Two. Three. Three fucking times. What are the odds of that? Even Google couldn't answer that for me.

My only remaining vice of sunbathing was now terminated, abruptly. I didn't drink, I didn't smoke. But I had had forty sessions of radiotherapy, which I'm sure was a contributing factor, as well as years of sunbathing both in and out of the UK. I just loved lying there feeling the heat on my body and watching the colour of my skin change from pale and washed out to bronzed and glowing. I, of course, Googled and Googled until I was an expert in the reasons, symptoms, treatments and outcomes for both of the skin patches, or to use the medical term, lesions.

Ian and I were in disagreement as to whether to tell the girls or not. He didn't want them to be worried. I didn't want to hold anything back from them and wanted to stick to my values of being open and honest. I also didn't want them to hear this from someone else. We agreed a compromise, that I would tell them the basics. Social and work lives prevented us all being together for forty-eight hours. It was hard to hold this news, as I felt I was being false when I was with them. I was nervous, and took a deep breath. I had rehearsed the words in my head. I told them an amalgamation of the basic facts from the GP and Google. I answered their questions in the same way. Poppy asked about the treatment and hair loss, twice. This was clearly playing on her mind. Who wants to tell their kids they have cancer? Not once, not twice, but three times. I felt I had let them down again. I felt I had failed to protect them again.

The following four days soon passed and I arrived at hospital number five. Based on what the GP had said, I would be okay. It would be a simple removal, and a low risk of more serious issues. After brief introductions, Dr Dermatologist was quick to swing into action and was soon pressing a large, illuminated, thick convex magnifying glass to my cheek, instantly pronouncing that the basal cell carcinoma diagnosed just four days earlier was in fact something else, which was benign. Relief.

She moved to the red chest patch thing and began exploring it in the same way. Dr Dermatologist announced some moments later that she didn't know what this was and therefore I would need a biopsy and this could be arranged for later in the day. WTF. I thought I would faint I was so stressed in that moment. I felt scared and out of control. How could this keep changing? How come four days ago this was nothing and now it was something and potentially serious; even she didn't know what it was. Where was my oncologist? He would have known, he would have told me there and then and come up with a plan, the delivery of a disaster mitigated with a plan of action and a serving of hope. I felt totally lost in those moments.

I was angry I wasn't being told. I questioned and questioned her, pushing for answers, something to hang onto in the chaos and uncertainty which had just hit me. My mind raced along the trajectory of skin cancers and possibilities, each with its own subtypes. Was it a basal cell? No. Was it a squamous cell? No. Was it a malignant melanoma? Maybe. I didn't recognise this one from the Google images stored in my mind and this was what the biopsy was going to determine. My anxiety went through the roof, ripping me away from the life and things I loved. My dignity departed rapidly. I was begging her to tell me. Now I had to tell the girls something else, a worse version of previous information. I worried their trust in me may waiver.

My anxiety and fear of the unknown triggered me to behave in a childish way at not getting the information I wanted, to return me to 'stage 1' (page 317) where I would feel safe again.

I used the time before the biopsy to familiarise myself with malignant melanoma images and any information available on Google. Malignant melanoma is a very different cancer to breast cancer and 1mm in tumour size can affect your survival possibilities enormously. This lesion was different; this lesion was red and not the traditional dark and irregular moles we associate with malignant melanoma and see on cancer campaigns. I carried on searching for pictures and understanding. Nothing matched or made sense. Finally I found a subtype of malignant melanoma called an amelanotic melanoma. This matched and made sense. My anxiety had something to focus on and attach to.

I began sending panicked texts updating friends and family. How could I do this to them again? I was stressed and distraught. I wanted safety and comfort, and yet knew no one could provide this for me.

Poppy was fantastic, seeing my struggle and said in a firm but calm and kind voice that if I didn't stop Googling she was going to take my phone away. I smiled inside at her care and sensible words. I was a tad embarrassed, but was also grateful she was parenting me. Ian was calm and said to wait for the results before I went to the darker places. Bonnie went about her day unphased by events.

I returned for the biopsy at the end of the clinic and apologised for my earlier expression of anxiety. As the biopsy preparation took place around me, I excused myself from any further conversation which would take place and began focusing solely on my breathing. In and out, deeply and rhythmically. Calm, calm, calm. If I kept breathing, I wouldn't faint. Scissors, tweezers, needles and thread moved in and on me. The following ten minutes were unpleasant but painless. I was stitched up and told I would receive the results by letter in two to three weeks' time. That sounded a long time, an unnecessarily long time to wonder if you had cancer or not, if you had a serious cancer or not. What would the treatment be? Would further tests be required? Had it spread?

I could not cope with any of what I had just been told or may have to face again. I could not focus on anything and my anxiety levels were huge. I feared the worst, imagining tumours growing silently in my liver and lungs. I'd been prepared for, and kind of expecting, a breast cancer recurrence. But skin cancer, I just didn't see that coming. I reflected that I had no regrets in my life because I had done so many amazing things, but I was so sad to think about having to let go of so much in the process of death, so many endings, so many goodbyes. I was terrified, paralysed with panic. I was morbid and morose. I was distracted and scared. My thoughts and fears consumed me. It was all I could think about all the time. Realisations came in torrents: the realisation of how hard dying must be, the realisation that I didn't think I could go through cancer again, the realisation of how hard I worked and struggled to stay positive and focused when I had spent twelve and a half years being terrified of dying of cancer, terrified at having to say goodbye to Poppy and Bonnie. For twelve and a half years I had worked hard to avoid these fears by living full-on and fast.

I felt instant 'trauma' (page 332) again with a further possible diagnosis, the unknown and uncertainty.

I struggled to hold my life together over the coming days. I wanted to tell people, to get rid of the thoughts and feelings, and yet knew they could not make this better. I just had to wait for the letter, and the words and diagnosis it would contain.

Day seven post-biopsy, someone somewhere would know something by now. But that someone wasn't me. By day nine the anxiety had increased to such a level that I was having panic attacks, sleepless nights and was struggling to hold myself together. I couldn't calm myself. Ian called Dr Dermatologist's secretary who confirmed the results were back, and Ian then imparted my mental state about not knowing what was happening. A couple of hours later, Dr Dermatologist kindly called and revealed the biopsy results. I wanted to hear, I wanted to know, but I also didn't; maybe if it was the bad type of bad news, not knowing was better. I couldn't breathe as she started to speak, my future and life held in her words. The biopsy showed I had the least serious of skin cancers, a superficial basal cell carcinoma. Breathe, breathe, breathe.

The treatment options were explained, my questions answered and I was booked in six days later to have the cancer frozen off or, to use the medical term, cryotherapy (a locally applied treatment where extreme cold in the form of liquid nitrogen is applied to the cancer, a scab forms and then falls off taking the dead cancer cells in it). Utter relief. Utter joy.

Just twenty-three days after seeing the Hugh Jackman Facebook post, the skin cancer was frozen off. No undressing or exposing, just the pulling down of my cold spring day layers. The cryotherapy felt like an icicle being inserted in to my skin, thin and piercing. The skin swelled and blistered. Leaflets were printed, detailing wound development and healing expectations, and a further appointment made for six weeks' time to see how the treatment had worked and, if not, the options available.

Done. I felt free to begin looking forward to a trip abroad we had planned over Easter where I hoped I could rest and relax, and soothe and switch off my mind, to escape cancer.

The site healed. We had our holiday. Vietnam was different and exotic. I was able to chill out and relax after the stress of cancer number three. I felt the white sand on my toes and the warmth on my skin. I looked at the blue skies and listened to the sea hour after hour, day after day, soothing my anxiety. I worked through my thoughts and feelings and thought about what I could change.

This skin cancer, although considerably quicker and easier to treat, and less serious than the previous two cancers, was every bit as traumatic, if not more so. I had not considered a different type and site of cancer. Cancer one taught me to live. Cancer two taught me to experience. Cancer three was now teaching me was how hard it is to live alongside cancer. The fear never quite leaves; ready to erupt again at the slightest trigger. How hard I had worked at being positive. How hard I had worked to protect others from the horror. How draining this all was and how I now needed to recognise this and change something. It was too much effort, too tiring, too exhausting to maintain this level of focus and concentration, to keep going, to keep cancer away from me and my life, and those who I love. I was constantly running, racing, escaping and hiding from cancer and death. Like a horrible game of chase where you know at some point you will be outwitted and caught, captured and unable to escape. This time I had no desire to go off and do something amazing. I was quite simply traumatised by cancer and living with cancer. Cancer was consuming my mind, if not my vital organs.

I had never admitted my struggles before. I hid my fears behind my smile, busy life and bucket list, but I could not go on doing that as it used too much time, energy and effort. And so I gave up the running. I would now just be. Accepting. It was cathartic, freeing and liberating to let go of this part of myself. The struggle had ended. Death would get me at some point and accepting that was better than constantly running from it.

The rest of the year passed and as 2016 drew to a close, I felt excited about 2017. I had let go of so much and I felt free. After considerable thought, I decided not to have a 2017 bucket list. They are tiring to achieve, to maintain focus on and to strive for. Their achievement occupied my mind and I ruled out other options in order to achieve them. Cancer and death have less of a hold on me now and so I don't need to focus on a bucket list to counteract these feelings and fears. In 2017 I decided to go with the flow and enjoy and make the most of what would come my way; less control and more spontaneity. For I had now accepted that I could not control or escape death.

CHAPTER 25

"It is the acceptance of death that has finally allowed me to choose life."

Elizabeth Lesser

had spent a blissful thirty-eight years, three months and eighteen days not thinking about death; it had never crossed my mind. However, once cancer came visiting I considered nothing else for a substantial amount of time.

Cancer forced me to think about death repeatedly; it kept clawing away in my mind. It was a long and at times painful process to make peace with this certainty of life. I am not scared about what happens after death but the process of dying does scare me. I assume I will die of cancer. I don't think about death via car crashes or heart attacks. I don't want to be in pain and I don't want to say goodbye to my gorgeous girls. Initially I thought that I would come back as a fairy and visit the girls on sunny summer days, hiding in the long grass watching them laugh and play.

By thinking about coming back as a fairy I was avoiding the finality of 'death' (page 321) and the permanent goodbye that it creates. I was 'bargaining' (page 326) that life would continue in another form.

Through therapy I gradually let go of the fairy scenario. It was difficult to think that I will die on my own and that no one can do this for me or with me. We do so much in our lives with other people, but death we have to face and experience on our own. As I faced my fears about death and separation from the girls, I began to recognise I held humanist views. Humanist views are based on the belief that we live just one life and there is no afterlife. The meaning to life is based on the choices we make and is not defined by society or theology. It is my responsibility to make my own decisions and create my own happiness and satisfaction.

By accepting the finality of life and letting go of the fairy scenario I was able to replace this with taking responsibility for creating a meaningful life.

The benefit of exploring and accepting death has been how I now live my life, and I am grateful that I have had time between my cancer diagnosis and death to live a meaningful life. I live every day as if it is my last. I don't take for granted I will be healthy tomorrow and know that one day I won't be. Each breath, mouthful, view or moment is appreciated and valued; there simply isn't time to waste or regret.

By recognising the finiteness of life, I make choices that are influenced by this fact. I ask myself daily what I want to achieve by the time I die. Death brought a stark clarity and focus to my life. Death reminds me of the life I want to lead. Death reminds me of the things I want in my life. Death reminds me of the things I don't want in my life. Death reminds me to focus on the significant meaningful stuff. I cannot avoid death, but I can live every moment of life meaningfully between now and then. At times this makes me selfish and tunnel-visioned.

Using the end of life as a filter to what I do and don't want in my life has created feelings of empowerment over death. This black and white, and at times inflexible and ruthless, 'configuration of self' (page 332) is in conflict with the softer, more caring 'configuration of self' (page 332). By living a meaningful life I have very little 'unfinished business' (page 331) and a daily gratitude and satisfaction in my life.

My biggest fear centred around dying when the girls were so young that they would not have a sense of who I was. Would they know I love fresh air, coastlines, woodlands, springtime, sunshine and wind? That my favourite flowers are lilies and my favourite food is fruit? That I loathe grey skies and rainy days? That I get excited about bluebell woods? That I hate offal and baked beans, and don't watch soaps? That my favourite number is the number 4? That my favourite birds are swallows? My sense was that Ian's pain of losing me would be too much and he would manage this by not talking about me. I was desperate that my memory was kept alive for the girls.

To create a sense of who I was, I started to write a daily diary of what we did and to collate a memory box of what we had done during each year. In the corner of the attic is a neat stack of brightly coloured A4 box files, each with the year clearly written on it, capturing and cataloguing memories. Each box is filled with mementoes and occasions: cinema tickets, train tickets, plane tickets, theme park tickets, school work, party invites, drawings and sketches, cute outfits, school awards and Christmas cards, handmade jewellery from pasta and painted shells, memories and love, in case I wasn't here to retell them. I hoped this would leave the girls with a sense of who I was as their mum and their childhood and that when they see a swallow or smell lilies they would remember me.

I didn't know if or for how long I would live and this created a huge fear and anxiety for me which was offset by being as proactive as I could in being the best mum I could be.

Poppy and Bonnie have been introduced to death via animals. I don't think this in anyway can prepare them for the death of a family member or friend, as the attachment and role they play in their lives and the ensuing absence will be different. I'm not sure how well I can prepare them for my death. I have told them I will be here for as long as I can be and that I would never choose to leave them. I have tried to make them independent and capable from an early age. We have talked about careers, wedding venues and a suitable partner to lose your virginity with, tattoos and drugs. I have tried to parent them for when I am no longer here. I have asked at my funeral that each person who comes writes a card about me, so the girls have something about me written by someone else, another perspective, thought or memory; the process of creating a bond with me for when I'm not here.

CHAPTER 26

*"If you really want to do something, you'll find a way.
If you don't, you'll find an excuse."*

Jim Rohn

That was my journey through three cancers in twelve and a half years. I would describe my relationship with cancer as complex. I can't quite hate it, because I wouldn't have achieved and experienced so much without it, but I can't love it either, with all the angst and upset it created. Cancer taught me many things, from how wonderful our NHS is, to appreciating the beauty of a sunrise. Cancer taught me that horrible things can happen to anyone at any time. Cancer taught me the value of time and to use it wisely. Cancer taught me I had resilience. Cancer taught me what pure fear feels like. Cancer taught me to live without regrets. Cancer taught me my strengths and weaknesses. Cancer took away my tolerance for what was not right in my life.

The cycle of anniversaries, tests, appointments, new registrars, treatments, traumas, triggers and feelings will continue. I am still traumatised by hospital appointments and what they may reveal and have found no way of managing those intense and overwhelming feelings. At times I act from a purely logical point and at times a purely emotional one. Cancer is not a linear illness with an endpoint. Cancer will remain an ongoing part of my life. I can never fully leave it behind and there will be dates and times where I will feel anxious and scared, but I have found a place to park cancer for today. Tomorrow may be different.

Struggling to overcome the inevitable and what I can't change is exhausting and futile, and I'm missing life in the process. I cannot avoid or outwit death; at some point I will have to face it, mine and others, the pain and destruction, the abyss of nothingness and grief which death creates. I have learnt to focus on what is, rather than what if, and to bring myself back to focus on what I have and not what I will lose. This helps me enjoy the here and now, and not what has happened or might happen.

Through cancer and the impact it has had on my life and relationships, I have faced many existential crises and traumas. The main loss was the certainty of life and facing the finiteness of life, which in turn led me to question and then revise the meaning of my life. From the dark places of isolation and fear came focus, hope, determination and then change. I live each and every moment with purpose and passion. Cancer triggered the expression of parts of myself which I liked, disliked or was unaware of. I worked out what nurtured me, what annoyed me and what needed to change in order to live a meaningful life and counteract the painful certainty of death.

Bargaining became a cancer coping strategy. Over the years I have become a professional bargainer, recognising what I can't change, and how I can empower myself with what I can. This helps me gain acceptance of each situation and frees me to live. In bargaining I can avoid my anger and possible injustice of what has happened, what has changed and been taken.

I recognised fairly early on in the world of cancer that no one was going to solve the situation or rescue me from it. I was on my own. Only I would be able to go to the appointments, hear the words, receive the treatments and recover. My oncologist became my safe and secure attachment figure in cancer. However, this created anxiety when he was unavailable. In my recovery I had to find what I wanted, what was safe and had meaning to me in the world, as I worked through Erikson's stages of development again to discover who I would be having had cancer. I felt like a teenager leaving home to find my way in the world once again.

My feelings of guilt and failure about being a good mum to Poppy and Bonnie have been difficult to accept. My idea of being a good mum was hugely damaged by cancer because I could not protect them from the impact cancer had on me, and that it took so much of my time and focus away from them. I have tried ever since to repair the unfinished business this created. As time has passed, I have put much in place for the girls; memories, trips, family times, life values and moral views. I have seen them and I have heard them. I have supported them in countless school and friendship issues, standing up for their views, needs and rights. I couldn't stand up for them in cancer, but I can for everything else. I feel I have done what I can do and set them on a solid path for life. As each year and milestone passes, I have appreciated the time we have been able to spend together. I feel I have now done a good job of being their mum and feel proud of who they are. The feelings of guilt and failure have eased as the girls have grown and are taking their steps out into the world. They are leaving me, I'm not leaving them before they are ready; the right order of things.

What kept me going through cancer was the drive to be there for my girls, and the belief and hope that I could do something to influence my future. I was able to focus on what I could influence and change, and in time accept what I couldn't. I learnt that when there was hope, I fought for what I wanted and this was triggered by the fight response.

I felt guilty for causing worry and concern to my friends and family with my cancer diagnosis and the risk to my life. To limit this distress, I now only tell them things that are concrete, the known and not the maybes. I stopped telling them the scares until they became facts, because I would worry them and feel embarrassed when I had to go back and say that actually it was okay.

The first time, cancer taught me to live. I was too angry and scared to enjoy life, which became rushed through at high speed and high octane. There was a drama at every corner and if I couldn't find one I created one. I became rebellious, selfish and took risks, each of which was a public and private 'fuck you' to cancer. It was an exhausting way to live.

The second time, cancer taught me to experience. Through practising mindfulness I learnt to savour life. I learnt to stop and experience moments, not rush past seeking excitement or creating the next drama. It was a quieter, calmer, less chaotic life, the drama and chaos replaced with satisfaction and stability.

The third time, cancer taught acceptance. I stopped running from death and the perpetual achieving. Death will eventually catch me. This acceptance has led to peace and calm. My feelings have been resolved and are now balanced and fluid.

I learnt when my feelings were overwhelming me and I couldn't tolerate or manage them, whether I felt anger or hopelessness, that I would channel them into an action; something else to focus on to counteract them. This is when the crazy ideas and bucket list were formed and they helped create hope, meaning and a way of reconnecting with life again.

Cancer took a great deal and taught me a great deal in the process; difficult but valuable learning which has led to a more satisfying life, wisdom which could not have been learnt in any other way.

PART II

THE IMPACT
FROM SOCIETY
ON CANCER

*"Progress is impossible without change
and those who cannot change their minds
cannot change anything."*

George Bernard Shaw

In this part of the book, I take a look at how cancer is portrayed and experienced in society, and how this impacts cancer patients.

CANCER LANGUAGE

The written and spoken word is an important and powerful communication tool across all areas of lives, cultures and nations. Language is used in different styles for different audiences; for example, the same news story may be covered in two different papers with both using different language to tell the same story, each with its audience in mind. Lawyers in a court case and teenagers arranging to meet their mates will all communicate in a way that has meaning to them. Cancer patients will probably have learnt a whole new language during their diagnosis and treatment.

Some of the words frequently used to describe cancer and cancer patients are: 'lost', 'battle', 'courage', 'brave', 'victim', 'beat', 'survivor' and 'fight'. Interesting, because if you ask a cancer patient about their experience of cancer, they are not generally words they would use and this difference can create a barrier when talking about cancer and therefore affect recovery. Cancer patients would probably tell you about their diagnosis and treatment, describing these using medical and pharmaceutical terminologies. They may also tell you about physical changes around hair loss, scarring or tiredness, and their emotions, such as sadness, depression, fear, hope, elation, powerlessness, hopelessness or anger.

Metaphors are important tools for creating mutual understanding and simplification of complex situations. For example, no one but me would know what my strained calf muscle felt like, but I might describe it as though I was being stabbed, or a fever as if I was on fire. Commonly the metaphors used to describe cancer are often based around war, implying winners and losers, victory and defeat. War-based metaphors may evoke motivation and empowerment in some, but disempowerment and failure in others, if a treatment is not working or a cancer is spreading, and they may stifle the important expression of negative feelings.

According to the media, I 'fought hard enough' that I became a cancer 'survivor'. What a load of rubbish. I was diagnosed and treated for cancer. I am not a victim or a survivor. I didn't do anything brave, I didn't have any fights and no battles took place. I wasn't attacked or injured. I didn't escape from a burning building or rescue a cat from a freezing mountainside wearing my slippers. Monuments are built and lyrics written about bravery, implying it has an aspect of choice about it. Cancer offers little choice. I had one choice; if I wanted to live I had to have the treatment and deal with the physical and emotional impact which occurred along the way. Cancer was not a battle, which I won, more of a storm that I had to face and do the best I could in.

While war metaphors may have their useful place to create unification, motivation and inspiration in fundraising campaigns they have little relevance to the individual and personal experience of cancer. They can create misunderstanding and separation when what a cancer patient really needs is empathy and connection. I prefer weather metaphors. Similar to cancer, the weather is powerful and out of my control.

War metaphors should be returned to battlefields and instead, terms describing cancer used. How about: 'diagnosed with cancer', 'affected by cancer', 'being treated for cancer', 'living with cancer', 'the experience of cancer', 'died from cancer', 'lost their life because of cancer'? These are informative and allow the individual's personal experience of cancer to be described and acknowledged.

There is hardly a day that passes without the media reporting a cancer-related feature: a death, a new treatment, or a food to eat or avoid. All too often a template of cancer clichés is used, with just a change of name, cancer type or outcome. Such articles become predictable and boring, sensationalist and insensitive. They speak loudly of the lack of understanding and effort of those who write, and bear little relation to the cancer experience. Would these words be used to describe other illnesses: heart attacks, strokes, multiple sclerosis, a sinus infection, diabetes, arthritis or flu? Probably not.

Media headlines prophesying cancer breakthroughs and 'cures' are common. These can misinform readers because it is only when you read the smaller text that you realise the drug may only be in the trial phase and is therefore probably many years away from large-scale use and potential benefit to extend lives. The use of the word 'survivor' also has issues in its meaning. If the word is used in a medical context, it will have a precise definition and criteria. How can you quantify a cancer survivor? One day, week, month or year after the end of treatment? Or is it dying of something else years later?

As diagnosis and treatments advance, surely the language and how we talk about cancer should too? Do these war words describe cancer for you or do you use them because everyone else does? Asking a cancer patient which words they would use to describe their cancer opens up the conversation, allowing them to talk about their unique experience in their own way. Choosing words that have meaning to them allows expression, creating empowerment and feeling understood, which will help their recovery.

CANCER CHARITIES

The NHS spends around £5 billion a year on cancer. However, the true cost of cancer is around £18 billion. This deficit is partially made up from the fundraising that cancer charities undertake. The work that cancer charities undertake is invaluable and has doubtlessly saved, sustained and extended countless lives. There are several hundred registered cancer charities in the UK alone, supporting: prevention to recovery; research to end-of-life care; young and old; male and female cancers; bereaved families; by cancer type and stage. Charities run on local, regional and national levels, each with a desire to help and support someone, somewhere; each needing funding to carry on their work. But how do some of the cancer charity slogans and campaigns impact and affect cancer patients?

The work that Cancer Research UK undertakes is vital and offers both support and information for cancer patients, and crucial funding to improve and develop cancer diagnosis and treatments. I have donated regularly for many years and have supported the charity many times. I have dressed top to toe in pink, penned and pinned heartfelt messages to my back and, along with Poppy and Bonnie, friends and family, taken part in countless Races for Life. I have also represented the charity as a media volunteer, spoken at a team-building event and taken part in a TV commercial.

It's a great charity and I passionately believe in the work they do. However, as a cancer patient, I struggle with some of the terminology used in their campaigns. I am frequently asked, generally in a cheery and hopeful manner, 'So you've got the all-clear?' I bristle and have to pause before I reply more realistically, 'I will never get the all-clear and I will always be at risk of a recurrence'. I have never heard any doctor ever say I have the 'all-clear'. I am classified as having 'no evidence of disease' on the day I have a test or check-up. One of their cancer campaigns suggested the 'all-clear' is permanent, and it's not until you delve a little deeper and into the smaller writing you discover 'all-clear' is defined as remaining cancer-free for five years after treatment.

Another Cancer Research UK campaign slogan quoted 'Let's beat cancer sooner'. I wondered how 'beat' and 'sooner' were defined? I contacted Cancer Research UK to ask for clarification. The reply I received was upbeat but evasive, and I'm left feeling the campaign is confusing without these words being defined.

The Pancreatic Cancer Action campaign, in February 2014, was based around a young female pancreatic cancer patient who stated, 'I wish I had breast cancer'. This caused many emotive responses. Delving a little below the surface, actually she wanted the survival statistics of breast cancer. The Pancreatic Cancer Research Fund cites statistics of progress in survival rates for other cancers, which feels like playing top trumps with cancer.

Some cancers do have better survival statistics and more treatment options. These tend to be cancers which develop in non-vital organs and are detected early through either self-discovery or screening. There is currently no life-extending screening test for pancreatic cancer and that is a harsh and difficult fact for pancreatic cancer patients and their loved ones.

Blood cancers were one of the earlier cancers where treatments were researched and developed, because the cancer could be seen in the blood. Trials, treatments and outcomes could be seen, monitored and adapted. Similarly, breast cancer has had decades of research and investment because it is growing in an area of our body that is not vital for our survival and therefore could be removed and researched. This feels unequal, and there is undoubtedly more treatment and hope for breast cancer patients.

However, metastatic breast cancer is a terminal illness from which there is no recovery. We should not forget that there are around 12,000 deaths a year in the UK alone from breast cancer, and that much has been learnt from treating this disease, which has been extended into other areas of oncology. Their suffering and death will be no less painful than others who have a cancer type that received less funding or a worse prognosis.

There is clearly a great need for cancer charities to continue the wonderful work they do and compete year-on-year for our attention and donations. They need emotive words and stories to do this. Fear and hope create this, but it is important to consider the impact campaigns have on the very people the charities are trying to help.

DEATH

Most people who have had cancer will have thought about death and dying, and a diagnosis of cancer may be the first time death has been thought about. Death is a complex topic and creates challenging thoughts to explore and reach some sort of personal conclusion, acceptance and peace about.

In the UK we don't like to talk about death and go to great lengths to avoid it. It is something that happens out of sight and preferably to other people. We become uncomfortable, awkward and embarrassed if the subject comes to close to us. But death will still happen regardless.

As healthcare has improved we have become more detached from death than previous generations. The reduction in exposure to death has increased our fears of it. Medical advances and research extends the boundaries of life on a daily basis, which has increased our expectations of living disease-free for longer, which can make talking about death even more difficult.

But not talking about death doesn't make it go away, it's still there and it will still happen. The impact is that when we do need to think about death it can be more difficult and the feelings more powerful because we have avoided talking about death.

In order for death to become part of life we need to have more day-to-day conversations about it. The more we think and talk about death the more we are able to accept it as a part of life. Talking about our fears of death can help the recovery of cancer and influence the lives we live because of it.

These are just a few of the issues cancer patients face in their lives and I hope that with awareness and time we can change some of these messages. Cancer cannot simply be described as a physical illness and its treatment and recovery need to reflect this.

THE WONDERFUL
WORLD OF
ONCOLOGY

"The good physician treats the disease;
the great physician treats the patient who has the disease."

William Osler

As a cancer patient you have no doubt had countless appointments, tests and treatments in a number of medical settings from numerous people. In this part of the book we will delve into that experience.

CANCER IN THE MEDICAL MODEL OF HEALTH

Cancer is predominantly diagnosed and treated in the medical model of health, which is the principal Western approach to illness and is influenced by science, finance and politics. The medical model primarily focuses on the physical and biological functioning of our bodies, in a clinical setting, where health is defined by the absence of a disease or injury, at which point we are discharged from the service; a world primarily based on a framework of facts, research, evidence, labelling, quantifiable measurement, cause, outcomes and a budget of billions of pounds. The process will usually include a presenting issue, taking a medical history, physical examination, tests (if needed), diagnosis, prognosis, treatment and a check-up, and this cycle may be repeated once or many times.

As we enter into this objective world, we are generally out of our knowledge and comfort zone, as we hand our lives over to be cared for by highly intelligent and skilled people who have many years of training behind them. In the medical model, the medic is seen as the expert and authoritarian who will follow a set of procedures with which the patient is compliant.

The impact of cancer triggers issues, thoughts and feelings which we probably have not encountered before, for which we need help and support to make sense of, manage and recover from. Although these may arise in and from the medical setting, there is not the time, support or budget to address them there. Unlike other illnesses, the needs of the patient continue long after the medical treatment has finished.

POST-CANCER TREATMENT NEEDS

Needs post-cancer are often left for cancer patients to work out, find, and probably fund, at a time when they may be feeling exhausted, vulnerable and fragile. It is this transition between the medical model, with its defined access and treatment paths, and discovering how to live with what has happened that can be challenging and leave a lasting impact on a cancer patient if they do not receive support during this period of adjustment. A cancer patient could be disease-free and therefore be seen as medically healthy, but not functioning in their life because they are recovering from the impact cancer has had on them.

TREATING CANCER HOLISTICALLY

A holistic model of care takes into account not only the physical needs of a patient, but also their psychological, social, emotional, environmental and spiritual wellbeing as well. This model of health moves beyond health being defined by the absence of disease, and suggests that health embraces all aspects of human experience, addresses the broader influences of health, and by nature will be as unique and individual as we are. The holistic model of health and care is less linear and aims to empower and enable patients to have active participation in their lives, improving emotional health, and creating and developing coping strategies, leading to a more satisfying life.

Holistic care can create emotional and psychological adjustment to diagnosis, treatment and recovery of cancer, thus reducing stress and distress. Some hospitals do offer this support, but it is not available everywhere and is more often found in the charitable sector locally rather than in a nationally available cancer recovery programme. Although costly to implement and maintain, the provision of this would reduce the huge financial impact cancer has on people personally, and the contribution we make to society. Surely it is time we moved towards an integrated healthcare system where emotional needs are treated with as much time, value and funding as our physical needs.

WHAT THE MEDICAL PROFESSION CAN DO

Working in the world of oncology is by nature challenging. We expect something different from an oncologist than we do from other relationships with other medical professionals, because we are vulnerable and in crisis, and potentially our life is at risk. Cancer brings something else out of us: our survival instinct, the drive to survive. Patients want oncologists to be warm, caring, committed and compassionate; they also want them to be capable and confident experts. There may also be an expectation that they meet, greet and interact with the patient's friends and family.

I'm sure it is extremely difficult to deliver the life-changing news of a cancer diagnosis and manage the world-crushing moments which follow. Each patient will have different needs. Some patients will want to know every detail, with an insatiable appetite for knowledge. Some will want to avoid as much as possible. Some will be comforted by a treatment plan and others will feel confined by it. Some will want a close relationship with their medical team, and others a more detached and distant one. This is all set within a framework of short appointment times; an emotionally charged setting; budget constraints; bulging clinics; balancing medical procedures, research and outcomes, and providing enough information to deliver an understanding and informed choice, but not adding to or triggering fear or trauma.

Doctors tend to be extremely good at assessing physical symptoms, but less so at emotional distress and psychological needs. The following are potential stress points for cancer patients during medical appointments and it can really help a cancer patient if they are minimised:

- Changing or conflicting advice
- Lack of choice, hope or time
- Discomfort at expressing emotions
- Medically directed and dominated appointments.

The following are helpful for cancer patients and reduce distress:

- Knowing the purpose of the appointment, test or treatment
- Clear and open communication
- Being prepared for the appointment, with test results and treatment options
- Checking the patient's subjective meaning of terminology
- Taking into account cultural needs, values and beliefs, as well as external influences in the patient's life

- Showing the patient you care about their physical and emotional health
- Consistency of staff
- Matching the patient's pace with the information you are giving
- Showing competence emotionally as well as medically
- Treading carefully on the thin line between hope and despair
- Allowing enough time for the patient's questions and emotions
- If you don't have the answers signposting to someone who does
- Looking for non-verbal communication cues, as well as what the patient is not saying.

As a cancer patient, trying to have your physical and emotional needs met in a medically dominated system can create frustration. It can be helpful to recognise where your needs will be better met in other locations. A compassionate, collaborative relationship with medical professionals can help reduce the debilitating effects of distress that cancer creates while treatment is taking place. The end of the active treatment for cancer can be a difficult time where cancer patients can feel abandoned by the medical world, and ideally support should be provided for this transition. Additionally, the emotional aspect of cancer recovery is vastly underfunded and underprovided for, which has a detrimental impact on a cancer patient's recovery.

WHAT HELPS THE RECOVERY FROM CANCER?

"May your choices reflect your hopes, not your fears."

Nelson Mandela

Being diagnosed with, and treated for, cancer permeates every part of our being and creates emotional and psychological issues affecting our relationships, sense of self and belonging. Cancer patients not only need physical care but also emotional care to recover from the impact cancer has.

Let's look in more detail at the impact that cancer has at each stage, from diagnosis through to recovery, and what may help with this.

DIAGNOSIS

Following a diagnosis of cancer, there will probably be a wide range of feelings: overwhelm, shock, disbelief, resentment, confusion, vulnerability, denial, anger, bargaining, fear, hope, stress, anxiety, sadness, depression, guilt, inquisitiveness, loneliness or relief. These feelings may be unfamiliar, and all of them are natural responses to a diagnosis of cancer, which for most of us can be defined as a trauma. Because planning for treatment, and the treatment itself, is likely to start quickly there may not be time to process these feelings before we become consumed with the practicalities and physical side effects of treatment.

There is inevitably distress around the time of diagnosis. There may be feelings of being out of control, with usual routines being disrupted and replaced with appointments, appointments and more appointments. There may also be a great deal of practical and logistical activity at this stage: planning for appointments and treatments, taking time off work, arranging childcare, or cancelling or rearranging commitments, plans or holidays. We start to replace the parts of our life that gave us meaning with treatment for cancer, and begin to experience the first losses cancer creates.

There may also be feelings of powerlessness. Feeling powerless is a major contributor to distress and, although the diagnosis and treatment can't change, there are times where choices can be made, which can create some autonomy. What are you in control of? What is out of your control? What can you achieve and take part in? What can you set aside for now?

There will probably also be feelings of fear about what lies ahead and the treatment. These feelings can be reduced by becoming involved with your treatment and engaging with the parts of your life that you enjoyed before the diagnosis, giving a sense of control and purpose. Although your life has changed in a dramatic way, you still have other areas in your life; don't forget about them, you are not just a cancer patient, defined by a diagnosis and treatment. Becoming involved with too much at this stage may be too challenging and overwhelming, but remember this for later when you feel ready.

When there is so much change, loss and uncertainty, it is important to hold onto hope for something, whether it's watching a movie with a friend, going on a favourite walk or planning a holiday at the end of your treatment. Find something you can look forward to achieving. What can you hope for today, tomorrow and next week?

Illness can make us vulnerable, passive and helpless. We may look for someone to help and support us, to resolve our distress. This can be challenging when we have probably been capable, autonomous adults for many years. A mismatch between support offered and support needed adds to a cancer patient's distress.

It can be helpful to look at what support you need and what you already have. This can be done by making a list of your needs and the resources (this can include friends, family, your strengths, what you enjoy doing) you have available. Then try to match the two, identifying areas of support and gaps in support.

Areas to think about:

- **Practical support**: What do you need for your appointments? Will you need help to get to and from them? Will you need to take time off work or to change your working arrangements? Do you want companionship or care while you are there or afterwards? Will you need practical support afterwards?
- **Emotional support:** Be as open as you can about how you feel and what you need. If you feel lonely, ask for contact. If you need to be alone, ask for time and space. What do you need in terms of emotional support? Who can you ask for help? Would professional support from your GP, support group or counsellor help? Earlier interventions are better than seeking support in a crisis.

Think about a typical day, week and month in your life. What do you need to do and what help might you need to complete these tasks? Offers of support tend to peak at diagnosis and steadily decline as time moves on and you may find it harder to ask for help in a few months' time. At times you are going to be physically less independent and your role in your life and that of others is going to change. My tip is to go with this and not fight it. Things will settle and in time your independence will return.

There is probably lots of information to share with lots of people. Take some time to think about how much information you want to share, with whom and when. An epic and uncontrollable game of Chinese whispers can quickly take hold and morph, with information being added and deleted as the story grows and evolves. I used social media, texts and emails as much as possible, so the written word was time-stamped and evidenced. The delivery of information via screens also helped because I didn't have to deal with initial reactions, tears, shock, platitudes or intrusive questions. People were able to express their initial response to the information before I saw them, which was less tiring and stressful for me.

Don't compare your diagnosis, treatment and outcome with anyone else's. Cancer is lonely and frightening at times, and you may want hope and reassurance from other people who have had a cancer diagnosis. Attaching to someone's experience of cancer in the short term may offer some relief, but in the long term it may be less helpful if your experiences become different.

TREATMENT

Treatment for cancer usually begins quite quickly. The treatment plan will often have been created by a team of several doctors and will aim to stop, slow down or eradicate the cancer. There may be complex drug names and treatments, with risks and side effects to understand and weigh up, as well as statistics and outcomes. There is often not time to fully work through the powerful feelings the diagnosis created before treatment begins, with most people muddling through or avoiding these feelings as they focus on the practicalities of the treatment which lies ahead and keeping their lives as stable as possible. However, these feelings do not go away; they remain unprocessed, unexpressed and unresolved.

During treatment, there are more than likely going to be some physical changes such as: scarring, shortened attention span, loss of movement, fatigue, weight gain or loss, or hair loss. These will also create emotional reactions. Feelings are likely to fluctuate and could be anything from positivity, relief, fear, sadness, happiness and anger, and maybe within the same minute. All these feelings are normal, expected and healthy reactions to the treatment and the impact it has. Feelings can be mild or intense, and it is important to be able to allow and express these feelings in a supportive environment.

Listen to what your body is saying to you. I found this very hard to do the first time around and would push myself past the point of exhaustion to avoid facing what was really going on. But if you listen to your body, it is really great at telling you what you need to do, rather than what you feel you should be doing. Second time around I did listen to my body and did as little as possible when I needed to. I saw my role as having the treatment and resting up to recover in the shortest amount of time possible. Look after yourself, and be kind and compassionate to yourself. Learn to check in with your feelings (physically and emotionally) on a regular basis. This may also help guide you on what you need.

Depending on the treatment you are having, you may have less energy and less time where you feel well, and time management may help to utilise this time. What do you need to do? What would you like to do? Prioritise and categorise everything by doing it, deleting it, delegating it or diarising it. The girls, running the home, work, family and friends were my priorities, and I spent my time and energy on these areas. It can also be helpful to recognise the times of day when you have more energy and prioritise your tasks accordingly.

It is important to spend some time doing activities which give you happiness and meaning when you feel well enough. Carrying on your life outside of being a cancer patient will keep you connected and less isolated.

It may be good to think about boundaries at this point. People dropping by unannounced can be well-meaning and have good intentions, but it could be inconvenient and put additional pressure or stress on you to entertain when all you may want to do is rest or cry. Questions about diagnosis, treatment and prognosis can quickly become overwhelming so again be prepared to put a boundary in about what you do and don't want to talk about. This can also apply to people offering tales of other cancer patients.

RECOVERY

So, the big day you have looked forward to, possibly for many months during arduous and difficult treatments, arrives; the day of your last treatment, the day you are no longer a cancer patient, the day you can return to your life without a schedule of appointments and a list of unpronounceable drugs to take. A happy day of relief and celebration? You'd like to think so, but it can also be a day of mixed feelings. You may feel happy, withdrawn, angry, vulnerable, depressed, anxious, disconnected, isolated or fearful. There may also be a loss of focus and purpose, as well as being fatigued beyond anything you have ever experienced.

Each person begins recovery from a different starting place. Take a couple of moments to notice what is going on for you. What are your thoughts and feelings about today? How has your life changed? What you have been through? What might happen next?

Every relationship and every part of your life will have been affected in some way by cancer. Whatever your thoughts and feelings at this time, they are necessary and normal, and part of the process of recovery will be to experience and express them. You may have held so much together for so long, just to get to this day, and there may now be time to reflect on the impact that the diagnosis and treatment had on you. Problems which were present before the diagnosis and may have been placed on hold while you focused on treatment may return now, adding to the turmoil. Additionally, the diagnosis and treatment may have triggered thoughts and feelings from the past. This can be a turbulent time while you process these thoughts and feelings, and can explain why people begin big projects at this stage as they search for a way to channel them and work out who they are in the world again after cancer.

The hospital appointments will probably end as abruptly as they began, which can leave you feeling lost and abandoned. There may be an expectation now that you've had your treatment, that your hair, smile, waistline and energy will return and you're good to go back to your life as it was. The mismatch in expectations (whether from ourselves or others) and reality can feel disappointing and pressurised. No one can see the emotional and psychological scars cancer creates, and these can remain long after the physical signs that you were a cancer patient have been covered over. Unfortunately, after such a life-changing event, things can never go back to exactly how they were and you may long for the seemingly innocent and carefree days where worries and troubles were focused on other areas of life.

The physical recovery from cancer often takes much longer than the treatment. Practically, do what you can do to minimise your physical recovery time. Eat well, exercise if you are able to and rest when you are tired. Allow your body time to recover. Nurture and nourish yourself. Take your meds as prescribed and attend any further hospital or screening appointments. Be kind to yourself and allow time for this process to take place. Regularly check in with yourself about how you are feeling physically.

Cancer can be described as trauma. When we experience a trauma, we are instantaneously helpless. A trauma wipes out our normal coping strategies and skills, and can challenge our feelings of trust and safety in the world. We only have a limited amount of brain capacity to manage trauma, and quickly become overloaded and overwhelmed. Following a trauma, we search for previous experiences to help ourselves and give us ideas or strategies to use to manage the trauma. If this fails, we search for someone to help us and, in some life events, we can succeed at this stage to stabilise ourselves again and move on.

There is no escape from a diagnosis of cancer; you can't pass it on to someone else or circumvent it, and you may feel you have no strategies to cope with the unknown that lies ahead in the short or long term. In order to move forward from the trauma and the impact it has had, you initially need to look backwards. Looking back can be daunting, as we naturally want to avoid connecting with the trauma.

Cancer is different from other traumas because it creates both acute and chronic trauma through diagnosis, treatment, recovery and ongoing life. Acute trauma may be intense and short-lived during diagnosis and treatment, while chronic trauma may create a cumulative effect through check-ups, screening and treatment side effects. It is these repeated exposures to the chronic trauma, coupled with the possibility of a recurrence that are difficult to adapt to because we can never quite leave cancer and its potential behind, with each test and appointment potentially triggering anxiety and fear.

To help you adjust to these changes, it can be beneficial to:

- Explore and express what has happened and how this has affected you
- Grieve for what you have lost or what has changed
- Find how the world can feel safe again
- Find purpose and meaning to your life.

It takes courage to speak out about how cancer affected and impacted on you, and may include facing fears and feelings of vulnerability and anger. However difficult this feels, exploring and expressing what has happened helps you to realise and work out how cancer affected you. You can achieve this in many ways and are in essence externalising your internal thoughts, feelings and turmoil. Talk about cancer every way you can: the diagnosis, treatment and recovery, your thoughts and feelings, and the physical impact too. Talk to family, friends or professionals.

Counselling is not for everyone, but it can be a supportive confidential space for this expression to take place in. There are also cancer support groups available both face-to-face and online.

If you find speaking the words challenging, you can also express what has happened to you creatively, through writing, art, music, poetry or dancing, or through objects such as shells, stones, buttons or photos. Noticing words, colours or bodily sensations, or having something to create or touch helps you to relate to your experiences, creating symbolic representations of our inner world, which in turn creates awareness, understanding and, in time, acceptance. Once you have acceptance, this allows you to move on and rebuild your life, which in turn builds your self-esteem and confidence, purpose, meaning and belonging.

It can be helpful, although potentially sad, to reflect on what has been lost or has changed by cancer. There may have been multiple losses, including: fertility, body parts, relationships, career, or life events. Again, it may be helpful to express this loss on our own or with other people. Loss never quite goes away, but we can live alongside it.

The world may feel unsafe following cancer, and part of recovery is feeling safe and secure again. However, as you have discovered, the world is full of unpredictable events that you have little if any control or influence over. As children, there is usually a caregiver to pick up the pieces and help you feel safe again. As adults, our relationships are different and no one can remove the unavoidable life event of death or the possibility of a cancer recurrence. This creates a dilemma of how to make the world safe again. As adults, we have to accept, balance and manage that at times we are going to feel threatened, but know where and how we can feel safe. Look for people, places or activities where you feel safe and trusting, and connect with those at times when you are feeling less safe.

Cancer is unpredictable. Feelings of safety tend to be temporary and need topping up because of the nature of the disease and the ongoing screening and appointments. Knowing and understanding as much as you can about your cancer, treatment and recovery, and being active in your treatment can help you feel empowered and safe. You may want to lead a quieter life following cancer and take fewer risks, which will add to a feeling of safety.

Once you have explored and expressed what has happened to you, what you have lost and how you can feel safe again, you will be more able emotionally and psychologically to reconnect with your life. When you feel ready, it can be helpful to set meaningful and achievable goals, broken down into bite-sized chunks, which will help you feel empowered. Setting and achieving goals can, in time, help restore confidence and self-esteem, as well as creating focus and hope for the future.

We crave a sense of belonging to groups of people, whether family, jobs, interests or friends. Social and human interactions are important for our emotional and psychological wellbeing. Cancer has more than likely affected this sense of belonging, because much has been changed by an illness which we find hard to talk about and understand and which takes us away from the sense of belonging that we may have spent years creating. The more you do, the more connected you will feel and the more you will feel you belong once more.

We cannot ever delete the trauma or potential for further trauma, but we can learn to manage our feelings relating to it. Trauma shatters our view of, and connection to, ourselves and others, creating disconnection and distrust, and a new, safe and meaningful world takes time to construct. Feeling connected and in control are important tasks during this stage of recovery.

Being treated for cancer takes us back to basics and what we need to do. Our lives can become simpler and, as a side effect, more enjoyable because there isn't the time or energy to spend on other stuff (stuff can be people, places, relationships, tasks or things), the stuff that drains us, the stuff we do out of a sense of duty, the stuff we do to avoid feeling guilty or rejected, or to please people. Take a moment to think what you would do if you could press pause on your life and start your life again. What would you take with you from your current life and what would you leave behind?

The end of your cancer treatment can be an opportunity for a mini (or major) life audit, de-junk or spring clean. Is there anything you would like to change? Is there anything you can change? How would you go about this change? Change is hard. Ending stuff is hard. But unless stuff makes you happy or adds something to your life, why would you have it in your life? Prioritise what makes you happy and what you care about, and work your way downwards; you will know when you reach the cut-off point as to what stuff doesn't make it back into your life, diary or to-do list. By doing this you will experience more peace and freedom, and less anxiety and irritation, together with a greater sense of purpose, meaning and satisfaction in life.

ONGOING

Unfortunately the impact of cancer doesn't always end once the treatment and recovery has taken place; now comes the lifelong task of living with what has happened. There is also the longer-term impact of the physical effects of treatment and any ongoing treatment, as well as managing the fear of a potential recurrence and the other emotions this creates.

Distress and powerful feelings are naturally high around a cancer diagnosis, but many patients continue to experience these from further referrals, screening, waits for results, anniversaries, and ongoing appointments and treatment. It is unsurprising that previous trauma is retriggered in situations when we feel under threat. Having consistent and trusting relationships with medical staff can help alleviate this.

We all seek safety, comfort and reassurance during times of anxiety and fear. My oncologist gave me reassurance with his knowledge and treatment plan, but I needed more frequent top-ups and I began to explore how else I could get this reassurance. I found myself asking my friends and family if I was going to be okay. Did they think the cancer was going to come back? As the words left my mouth, I realised I was being both unfair and unrealistic, but that is how anxious I was. I began to recognise that, in asking this question, there was the potential for rescuing and giving me the answer they felt I wanted to hear. I began endless Google searches. That didn't work either, so I went back to the facts, the medical facts. The medical facts were that I had had a clear CT scan and a clear bone scan. My oncologist had said there was no reason why I couldn't have another ten years and Mr Radiologist had said that cancer rarely returns to an area that has been treated with radiation. I had no symptoms and I still have no symptoms. I feel and look well. I keep this as an anchor when my mind takes a trip to anxiety freak-out fantasy funeral land. I check in with myself physically and if I'm okay, I get on with living.

What reassurance was I seeking? I was seeking the impossible: that I wasn't going to die. I was seeking external sources to soothe my internal fears, which was never going to work in the short or long term. Instead of seeking reassurance for something that is definitely going to happen, I have instead worked on accepting my death *will* happen and by living my life, which has reduced my need for reassurance. What are you seeking reassurance for and why? Who or what can give you this reassurance? How long does the reassurance last for? Do you notice when your fear or anxiety reappears?

Life after a cancer diagnosis requires resilience, because previous trauma and distress can be retriggered. Resilience is the subjective process of adaption and recovery from adversity. We may also react differently to the same adversity should we experience it more than once. When the adversity is too great, our resilience becomes overwhelmed and we are left feeling distressed.

As with other personality traits, some people are born with more resilience than others, or are able to use it more effectively. It does not mean that these people don't feel distress at adversity; it means that they are able to adapt to the situation better than others. Although external factors can influence resilience, ultimately this has to be driven internally, from within ourselves. Research shows that we can build resilience and therefore how we respond and adjust to adversity. Factors include having loving, caring, supportive and trusting relationships; a positive view of ourselves; an awareness of our abilities and strengths; the ability to manage strong feelings; the ability to be able to make and carry out plans and goals, and resolve problems; the ability to accept that change and adversity is an unavoidable and unchangeable part of life; the belief that we can move beyond the adversity to achieve our goals; and self-confidence.

There are many events in life which we can't control – the weather, traffic jams, other people, football scores or illness. Trying to control the uncontrollable is both futile and soul-destroying, and we are left frustrated when we try to do so and can't. We can't control a diagnosis of cancer, we can't control the path of the disease and we can't control our response to treatment. It is during these events, which we have no control over, that it is important to seek some aspect of choice, because it provides us with a sense of control and safety.

There are life events which we can influence and control: jobs, relationships, where we live, where we travel, what we eat, as well as the thousands of choices we make on a daily basis. Spending our time, energy and focus on what we can control and influence, will lead to less anxiety, less stress and greater life satisfaction. In time, and with practice, this becomes a grounding way of living; life becomes simpler because we invest more time and energy into what we can control and influence.

I have learnt that I can't choose the cards I'm given, but I can control how I play them. The fact that I have had cancer, that I may have cancer again and that I'm going to die are all out of my control; I acknowledge them, but don't dwell on them. I don't believe I can 'beat' cancer and, therefore, I'm focused on living as much life as I can, as well as I can, for as long as I can.

Although the recovery from the diagnosis of and treatment for cancer can be a difficult and complex time, it can also be a time for deep change and rich reflection, a chance to pause and assess your life after the storm. You probably won't get all the answers by the end of day one, or day two for that matter; change takes time. I cannot give you the magic answer or formula for recovery from cancer, but I can give you a framework and areas to look at.

Recovery is neither a competition nor a race to the finish line. Trust your instincts and listen to what your mind and body are telling you, trust what is right for you, and listen to others but trust yourself, as only you have to live your life and your recovery within it. Only you can experience and process your thoughts and feelings, and how they affected and impacted you.

THE END

*"We must pass through our own shadows
before we can emerge into the light."*

Carl Jung

I hope this book has helped create understanding about the impact that cancer has. I hope this book has helped your recovery from cancer. I hope this book has inspired you to live your life fully. I hope this book gives you hope that you can overcome adversity. I hope that, having read this, you can change something for a cancer patient you may know, meet or become.

You will find a way to get through the treatment and trauma of cancer, and in time rebuild your life. It will be difficult and it will be a different life, and in that process you will learn, fail and, I hope, try again. Please don't underestimate the enormity of what you have been through and that this will change who you are and possibly who you want to be. Remind yourself of what is and isn't in your control, focusing your time and energy on what you can control and influence, and work on what you may need to accept.

People frequently say they feel sorry for me living with cancer; I feel sorry for people who aren't living. Make every moment and every choice count. I learnt that through the chaos and change caused by one tiny cell.

COUNSELLING THEORY

"The most creative act you will ever undertake
is the act of creating yourself."

Deepak Chopra

This part of the book gives an overview of the counselling theory I use to explain my experience of cancer, which I hope will create a greater understanding of what it is like to have cancer. There is no need to read this section in full (unless you want to); I will refer to the relevant pages at various points throughout the book. There are more detailed explanations of these theories on the internet, and many published articles and books, but for this book I aim to keep things simple.

It's probably good to look at what counselling is before I start explaining some of the theory which underpins the techniques and interventions I use in my work with clients. Counselling is a type of talking therapy that allows a person to talk about their problems, thoughts, behaviour and feelings in a confidential and dependable environment with a trained counsellor. Counselling can help you gain awareness and understanding, and identify changes you can make, empowering you to find solutions.

There are a vast number of counselling models, concepts and interventions. My counselling training focused on the humanistic models and ethos. These models are based on the belief that we are all unique individuals with the potential and capacity to grow and develop throughout our lives. By taking responsibility for our thoughts and actions, and through increased awareness, we can make better choices, leading to a more satisfying, autonomous life with greater personal fulfilment. Humanistic therapy focuses on the dynamic self in relation to the current environment we are in. It looks at the person as a whole rather than a particular thought, feeling, behaviour, or part or period of life, and therefore differs from behavioural and psychoanalytical models of counselling.

ATTACHMENT THEORY

I will begin with attachment theory because that is where we all begin really. Attachment can be described as an emotional bond to someone else. John Bowlby's research (1988, A secure base: Parent-child attachment and healthy human development.) suggested we have an instinctive and lifelong need for attachments to other people, because as mammals our survival is dependent on them. Attachments are formed early in life through our primary caregivers' response to our needs. This goes on to influence how we form and relate in future relationships, based on trust of others and ourselves. We can become attached to a variety of things; people, places or animals. If a child's needs are not met with sensitive and consistent attunement, the child develops strategies to manage their needs within the caregiver relationship and subsequent relationships.

A child seeks protection, comfort, safety and security when they feel scared, ill or tired. When they feel safe again they return to exploring the world knowing and trusting they can return when needed. These feelings continue into adulthood, where we may ask a partner or friend to protect or comfort us at times of difficulty until we feel safe again. Mary Ainsworth's (1985, Patterns of Attachment.) research identified different styles of attachment depending on the coping strategy developed if there was unresponsive caregiving.

SECURE ATTACHMENT

When a primary caregiver provides sensitive, flexible and responsive care, we form a secure attachment with them. A secure attachment creates a greater sense of self-esteem as well as trust in other people, and comfort with both intimacy and independence.

AVOIDANT ATTACHMENT

Those who form an avoidant attachment tend to avoid intimate and close relationships, and seek independence because the caregiving they received was consistently rejecting or unavailable.

INSECURE ATTACHMENT

Those with an insecure attachment tend to seek approval and reassurance in relationships and can become demanding and clingy, and display anxiety if this is not received. The care they received was unreliable or inconsistent.

ERIKSON'S STAGES OF DEVELOPMENT

Erik Erikson (1959, Identity and the life cycle.) proposed a model of development which spans a lifetime from infancy to late adulthood, with each stage building on the previous one. The eight stages take into account the conflict between the psychological and social needs of the individual. Successful resolution of the crisis in each stage creates a healthy personality with the ability to resolve future crises.

Stage 1 (0 to 18 months) Trust vs mistrust. This stage explores the crisis of whether the world is a safe place or not. The infant looks to the caregiver for consistent care to counteract the feelings of uncertainty. This helps them to feel safe, develop trust and sense of security, and have hope that in future crises there will be support available. If hope is not acquired, anxiety and fear will develop.

Stage 2 (18 months to 3 years) Autonomy vs shame and doubt. During this stage, children begin to assert their independence and make choices, discovering their skills and limits in ability. They also begin to take care of their basic needs such as feeding and dressing themselves. Parental encouragement is needed to help develop their autonomy, as well as to provide support when failure inevitably occurs. This helps to create confidence and develop self-esteem. Success at this stage leads to will; if will is not acquired, a child may doubt their abilities.

Stage 3 (3 to 5 years) Initiative vs guilt. During these lively years, children develop rapidly. Through regular interaction with other children via play, where interpersonal skills are explored and practised, children can foster a sense of initiative and decision-making. If this initiative is controlled or criticised, a sense of guilt can develop and children remain followers, lacking creativity, and they may feel guilty for being a nuisance. Success at this stage leads to a sense of purpose.

Stage 4 (5 to 12 years) Industry vs inferiority. During this stage, a child's peers and teachers will become of greater significance to a child as they learn new skills. They gain pride in their accomplishments and in turn feel valued, which builds their self-esteem. If children receive encouragement to achieve their goals, they begin to gain confidence. If children are restricted at this stage, the child feels inferior, doubting their abilities. If they are unable to develop a specific skill that they feel society values, e.g. a dyslexic struggling to read, they may develop a sense of inferiority. Success at this stage leads to a sense of competence.

Stage 5 (12 to 18 years) Identity vs role confusion. This stage covers the transition from childhood to adulthood. Children become increasingly independent and begin to focus on their future, such as careers and relationships. They also begin to think about how they will fit into society as well as the roles they will fulfil in adulthood. During this stage, the adolescent will try to find out who they are by trying different roles out, including their sexual self and body image. By trying these roles and experiencing the outcomes, they form their identity. Success in this stage will create self-esteem and confidence. Failure at this stage leads to role confusion of self and within society.

Stage 6 (18 to 40 years) Intimacy vs isolation. During this stage, we begin more intimate, longer-term, safe and committed relationships. Avoiding these can lead to isolation and loneliness. Success in this stage leads to love.

Stage 7 (40 to 65 years) Generativity vs stagnation. During this stage, careers and families are established. We give back to society through, for example, raising children, our careers and community projects. Failure at this stage can lead to feeling stagnant and unproductive, whereas success leads to the virtue of care.

Stage 8 (65 years and over) Ego vs despair. As we grow older we slow down and explore life as a retired person. There may be more time to contemplate our accomplishments, developing integrity if we reflect that we have led a successful life. If we view our lives as unproductive or we did not achieve our goals or feel guilty about our past or have regrets, we can experience despair, depression and hopelessness. This can be a very rich part of life if we have led a satisfying life or have felt able to make changes to feel satisfied. If we are not able to make changes, this stage of life can be difficult, when we are aware of our finiteness but also feel powerless to make a change. Success at this stage will lead to wisdom and reflection with a sense of completeness.

That is a very brief tour of one theory of how we develop. Let's now look at the boundaries of our existence, which is a little heavy going.

EXISTENTIAL PHILOSOPHY

Existential philosophy has been written about for centuries and focuses on our existence and what it means to be human. We all live with four aspects of our existence which we cannot choose: we are born; where we are born; our gender and race; and we are going to die. These facts are unchangeable. Existential anxiety can arise if people contemplate their existence at a deeper level. However, unlike fear and anxiety, with existential anxiety no specific danger presents itself. If people explore who they are, where they belong or what their purpose in life is, this creates awareness of the existential givens and a sense of dread around isolation, purpose and death.

Existential philosophy is based on the premise that despite the external expectations of the roles we have in life and the culture we live in, we are independent individuals who have freedom and choice. It becomes our responsibility to create value and meaning in our lives and to live authentically. In that process we will falter and fail, risk rejection, and experience illness, hardship, doubt and despair.

EXISTENTIAL GIVENS

Existential philosophy also explores our inner conflict due to confrontation with four unsolvable facts of life – death, isolation, freedom and the meaning of our existence – which affect us all; these are known as the existential givens. We are more likely to experience the givens during times of life changes and transitions. However, experiencing, processing and accepting the givens creates an opportunity to lead an authentic life. An authentic life is achieved through making choices, and balancing possibilities and limitations by being aware of the givens but not overwhelmed by them. Because the givens are difficult to experience, we develop strategies to avoid them, such as focusing on our work, making money, being youthful, relationships, alcohol or exercise. But, however hard we try, the givens are impossible to remove and the strategies we adopt to avoid them require increasing amounts of time and energy to maintain.

EXISTENTIAL GIVEN OF DEATH

The given of death focuses on the temporality of our existence and that we are inevitably going to suffer loss and die. Many of our anxieties are created from the fear of death and our avoidance of it. However, if we fully embrace death and the finiteness of our existence it can help us make better choices and can influence the meaning we choose for our life. Most people are unlikely to engage with these thoughts through choice and only do so when forced to, maybe through age or illness. We avoid, and counteract engaging with, thoughts and feelings around death by leading a busy life, imagining a peaceful death or having a belief in the afterlife.

EXISTENTIAL GIVEN OF ISOLATION

The given of isolation explores our experience of isolation and loneliness. We are individuals and no matter how close we feel to people, we are still separate. We enter, suffer and leave the world on our own; no one can live these life events for us.

EXISTENTIAL GIVEN OF FREEDOM

The given of freedom explores that we are entirely responsible for our lives. We are free to take responsibility, make choices and experience the consequences.

EXISTENTIAL GIVEN OF MEANING

The given of meaning centres around the individual meaning of our existence. We are born into a world which has no set meaning. If our life has no meaning or purpose we can feel hopelessness.

Existential philosophy also takes into account that we each relate to, and encounter, the world subjectively and experience the givens through four different dimensions of existence which interact and intertwine, creating our individual reality.

PHYSICAL DIMENSION

The physical dimension (the given of death) is our relation to the environment and surroundings in which we live. This includes nature, our bodies, material possessions and our health. Our physical existence begins with birth and ends with death. We struggle and strive to feel dominant over things which are impossible to have dominance over. In an attempt to counteract these feelings, we seek to create security, but this can only be achieved temporarily as our mortality is an unsolvable dilemma which we can either embrace or deny. Everything in our lives is temporary: health, wealth and happiness.

SOCIAL DIMENSION

The social dimension (the given of isolation) is how we connect, relate and interact with the public world around us. This includes our responses to culture, race and class, and what we do and don't belong to. We may sacrifice our needs in order to fit in with expectations and rules of others to avoid facing the fear of isolation and rejection from others. Our unsolvable dilemma in this dimension is around retaining our individuality, but also needing to be connected to others for our physical and emotional survival because relationships are unavoidable.

PERSONAL DIMENSION

The personal dimension (the given of freedom) creates our internal, personal view of the world. This will include our character, strengths and weaknesses, as well as our past experiences and potential possibilities, all of which contribute to creating our sense of identity. However, events will constantly challenge and change these views, during which we will experience loss of self and we will seek a revised view of the world. During this process we realise that we have freedom to make choices and take responsibility for our actions. This process develops personal strength as we have to live with the consequences of our actions. Distress is caused by not taking responsibility for the things we do have responsibility for, as well as taking responsibility for things we don't have responsibility for.

SPIRITUAL DIMENSION

The spiritual dimension (the given of meaning) relates to the unknown. This dimension explores creating an ideological and philosophical view about the meaning of the world and our attitude to life. This could be achieved through religion or in a secular way creating value in something. We may face feelings around hope and despair as we strive to create something of value to avoid facing nothingness in our lives. The dilemma in this dimension is recognising that there is no universal system of value and we need to create our own meaning, purpose and values.

EXISTENTIAL CRISIS

At some point in our lives we may experience an existential crisis. An existential crisis is often provoked by a significant life event such as divorce, job loss, children leaving home or a life-threatening illness such as cancer. It becomes a time when we question the meaning, purpose and values we have in our lives. Although difficult to experience, an existential crisis can be an opportunity to review and rebuild meaning and purpose in life.

Existential stuff is quite challenging and possibly confusing, and I'm sorry but the next theory is no lighter; these all form a large part of the emotional and psychological impact cancer has on us.

LOSS

There are many models of the theory about loss and grief, but the one I work with most frequently is that of Elizabeth Kubler-Ross. Through her work with the dying, Kubler-Ross identified five stages of emotional reaction to a loss (denial, anger, bargaining, depression and acceptance), which can be applied to any loss. The stages are described in a linear way, but may not be experienced in this sequence. People can spend different amounts of time in each stage or get stuck in one. Feelings may be experienced with differing intensity in the different stages and people may return to a stage several times before reaching acceptance. There is no right or wrong way to grieve, but resisting or avoiding engagement with the feelings ultimately prevents us from accepting the loss.

DENIAL

Denial is a first and temporary reaction to overwhelming feelings and facts. Denial acts as a defence to protect us from the immediate shock of the loss and allows us time to absorb and rationalise the information.

ANGER

Anger can be experienced as the masking effect of denial fades. We realise the denial cannot continue and reality begins to emerge as we realise the loss is happening. Anger can manifest itself in many ways and we may look to blame someone or something such as doctors, our faith, family or ourselves. Anger acts like an anchor keeping us attached to what we have lost, and underneath this anger is often pain.

BARGAINING

Bargaining is an attempt to postpone the inevitable and manage our vulnerability by negotiation and reform, providing us with a sense of feeling in control and creating hope. We can also feel guilty during this stage and wonder 'What if?' or 'If only I had'.

DEPRESSION

Depression is experienced when we realise that bargaining

is not going to work and we become aware of the loss we face and what this means to us. The previous stages are located in the past but depression is in the present.

ACCEPTANCE

Acceptance is when we begin to accept the situation is not going to go away. This can be a period of calm. This may not happen to everyone as we may get stuck in an earlier stage, especially if the loss is sudden. We can never replace what we have lost, but we can make new connections, change and grow.

TRANSACTIONAL ANALYSIS

Transactional Analysis is a model of counselling which explores interactions and communication with others. It was developed by Eric Berne in the 1950s. Transactional Analysis aims to improve communication with others through awareness and changing dysfunctional communications.

DRAMA TRIANGLE

One concept used in Transactional Analysis is the Karpman Drama Triangle which was written about by Stephen Karpman in 1968. The concept suggests that people take three roles in a situation (often unconsciously and starting in childhood): victim, persecutor and rescuer. These roles lead to dysfunctional communications through conflict of power and responsibility. Each role eventually leads to frustration, retaliation and a rotation in roles, i.e. the victim becomes the persecutor.

VICTIM

The victim is vulnerable, helpless or hopeless, and often denies or avoids taking responsibility.

PERSECUTOR

The persecutor uses power, criticism, pressure, blame, coercion or control to have their needs met, often at the victim's expense.

RESCUER

The rescuer takes responsibility and views the victim as vulnerable in some way. The rescuer intervenes with a desire to help the victim, but may in doing so, have their needs met, i.e. by raising their self-esteem and creating dependency.

DRIVERS

Another concept in Transactional Analysis is Drivers. Drivers were identified by Taibi Kahler in 1975 and describe the unconscious internal pressures which motivate us to achieve in certain ways. Drivers satisfy inner needs rather than responding to the external event they are relating to. Drivers can therefore become dysfunctional behaviours causing stress and further dysfunctional behaviour in an attempt to mitigate the feelings they create. Drivers are often learnt in childhood to seek approval and can influence our thoughts, feelings and behaviours later in life.

BE PERFECT

The 'be perfect' driver displays behaviour which must be perfect and correct in every way, as well as achieve success in everything which is done. People with this driver are hardworking and the quality of their work is excellent and often without mistakes. There is a fear of failure and loss of control, as well as expecting others to be perfect too, displaying little compromise.

BE STRONG

The 'be strong' driver displays behaviour which must not be vulnerable or show weakness at any time. The attitude is often assertive or aggressive to demonstrate strength. This driver is good for getting tasks done, especially in a crisis; however, the bottled up emotions can explode out towards others. There may also be an expectation of others to be strong, and contempt for the weak.

TRY HARDER

The 'try harder' driver is where we are never satisfied with what we have achieved and can always do better. Satisfaction is rarely experienced at what has been achieved, despite having given our utmost. Praise is craved but does not satisfy when received. Criticism is very hurtful to people with this driver and there is an expectation that others should try harder too.

PLEASE OTHERS

The 'please others' driver is where we do things to please others and feel we must make them happy. Thoughts can include those of 'only others can tell me when I have done well' and 'if they don't I have failed'. This driver seeks approval and is easily offended.

HURRY UP

The 'hurry up' driver is where everything has to be done at speed; there is much to do and not much time to do it in. This driver creates enthusiasm as well as impatience and frustration. The focus and delivery is action-orientated with good output.

GESTALT THERAPY

Gestalt Therapy is a form of counselling which was developed in the 1940s by Fritz Perls. The basic principles in Gestalt Therapy are that the individual is treated as a whole, taking into account the mind, body and soul, and that people are best understood in relation to their unique and current situation and environment and their experience of it. The theory focuses on the here and now, increasing self-awareness around negative thoughts and patterns of behaviour which can lead people to feel unsatisfied and unhappy. It also explores the theory that in seeking to have our needs met we develop patterns of behaviour which we may not be aware of.

UNFINISHED BUSINESS

A concept within Gestalt Therapy is that unfinished business (tasks and goals that we want to achieve, the expression of feelings or resolution of unresolved issues) creates anxiety, grief, anger and a sense of preoccupation which lingers with us until it is completed. These feelings associated with unfinished business can originate from many years ago.

PERSON-CENTRED THERAPY

Carl Rogers was the founder of Person-Centred Therapy in the 1950s. Person-Centred Therapy focuses on how a person views themselves and this can be influenced by internalising messages from others. The counsellor explores a person's experiences from their point of view and, in the process, creates awareness, understanding and choice.

SELF-ACTUALISATION

Rogers suggests we all have an inner drive to reach our full potential, no matter what the conditions are (think of potato shoots growing in a dark shed towards sunlight). This is known as self-actualisation. Self-actualisation drives desire for something better in our lives, such as getting a job or learning to paint. The need for personal growth and development remains throughout our lives.

CONFIGURATIONS OF SELF

Another concept in Person-Centred Theory is known as configurations of self. Configurations of self are adaptions of ourselves used to relate to, and even survive in, a variety of circumstances. Think about yourself at work and then on a night out with your friends. I doubt you behave the same in both situations. Some of these configurations may seem contradictory and can trigger both positive and negative emotions and behaviours.

I will also refer to the following terms:

TRAUMA

A trauma or traumatic event can be described as an overwhelming event that we have no control over, which we cannot avoid and which we have no known ability to cope with. A trauma can be an event that causes physical, emotional or psychological harm and could be an accident, violence, death or natural disaster, or disease such as cancer.

LOGICAL AND EMOTIONAL RESPONSES

Our brains use both logic and emotion to inform and guide us. We make thousands of choices each day, from where to sit on the sofa to when to cross the road. Our brains are constantly balancing the logical and emotional responses from the information we receive through our senses. If we respond from only one part, the outcome is usually short term because it is unbalanced. Our best choices and responses are when we integrate both logic and emotion. Sometimes we react quickly and wholly from one point. People who are not aware of their feelings, or find it hard to experience or express them, may respond very logically, whereas people who are very emotional, and at times helpless and reliant on others, may need to be more engaged with their logical brain and recognise their capability and responsibility.

IN CONTROL, OUT OF CONTROL, INFLUENCE

Life and life events fall into three categories: those we can control, those we can influence, and those we can't control. We all have a need to feel in control of our environment and lives; this originates from an evolutionary position of survival. If we are in control of our surroundings we have an increased chance of survival. If we don't feel in control we may not feel safe and this can create potent and uncomfortable feelings of powerlessness, which in turn can create feelings of anger, triggering the 'flight, fight, freeze or flop' response to the perceived danger.